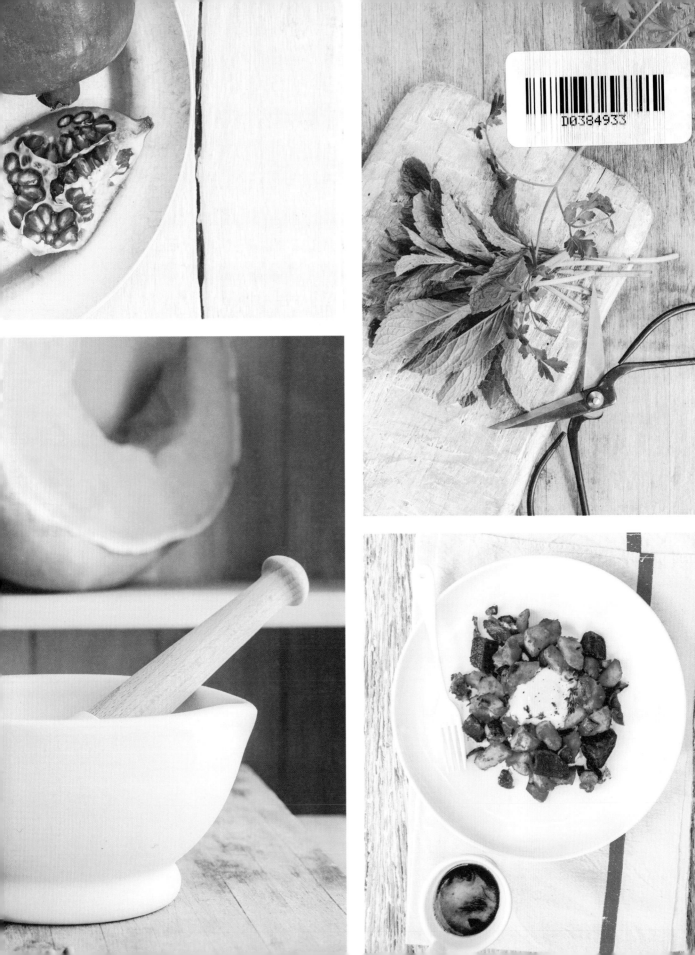

The
Superfood
KITCHEN

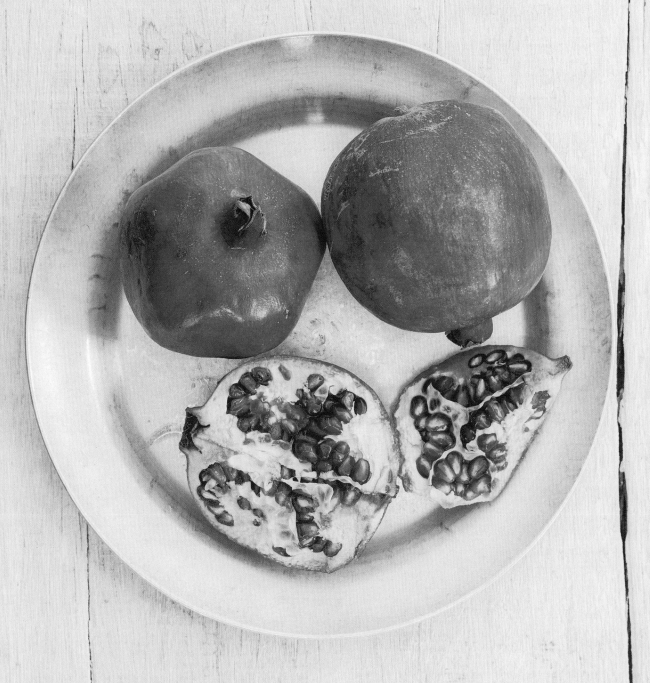

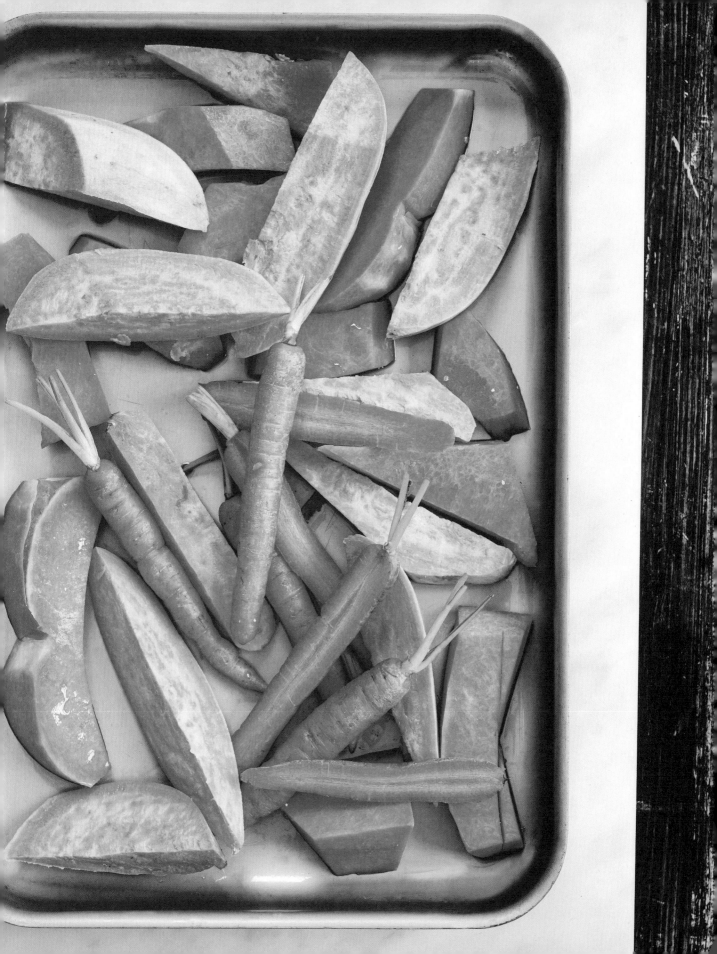

The Superfood

KITCHEN

This edition published by Parragon Books Ltd in 2014 and distributed by

Parragon Inc.
440 Park Avenue South, 13th Floor
New York, NY 10016
www.parragon.com/lovefood

LOVE FOOD is an imprint of Parragon Books Ltd

Copyright © Parragon Books Ltd 2014

LOVE FOOD and the accompanying heart device is a registered trademark of Parragon Books Ltd in the USA, the UK, Australia, India, and the EU.

ISBN: 978-1-4723-6455-5

Printed in China

New recipes and food styling by Sara Lewis
Created and produced by Pene Parker and Becca Spry
New photography by Haarala Hamilton

Notes for the reader

This book uses standard kitchen measuring spoons and cups. All spoon and cup measurements are level unless otherwise indicated. Unless otherwise stated, milk is assumed to be whole, eggs are large, individual vegetables are medium, and pepper is freshly ground black pepper. Unless otherwise stated, all root vegetables should be peeled prior to using.

Garnishes, decorations, and serving suggestions are all optional and not necessarily included in the recipe ingredients or method. Any optional ingredients and seasoning to taste are not included in the nutritional analysis. The times given are only an approximate guide. Preparation times differ according to the techniques used by different people and the cooking times may also vary from those given. Optional ingredients, variations, or serving suggestions have not been included in the time calculations.

Where the author has made all reasonable efforts to ensure that the information contained in this book is accurate and up to date at the time of publication, anyone reading this book should note the following important points:

* Medical and pharmaceutical knowledge is constantly changing and the author and the publisher cannot and do not guarantee the accuracy or appropriateness of the contents of this book;
* In any event, this book is not intended to be, and should not be relied upon, as a substitute for advice from your healthcare practitioner before making any major dietary changes;
* Food Allergy Disclaimer: The author and the publisher are not responsible for any adverse reactions to the recipes contained herein.
* The statements in this book have not been evaluated by the U.S. Food and Drug Administration. This book is not intended to treat, cure, or prevent any disease.

For the reasons set out above, and to the fullest extent permitted by law, the author and the publisher: (i) cannot and do not accept any legal duty of care or responsibility in relation to the accuracy of appropriateness of the contents of this book, even where expressed as "advice" or using other words to this effect; and (ii) disclaim any liability, loss, damage, or risk that may be claimed or incurred as a consequence – directly or indirectly – of the use and/or application of any of the contents of this book.

CONTENTS

Introduction 6

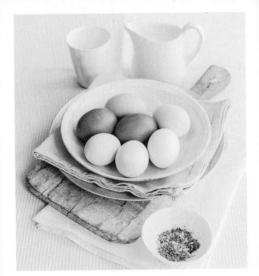

Breakfasts 18

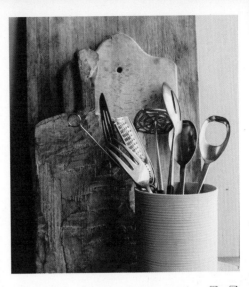

Lunches and snacks 44

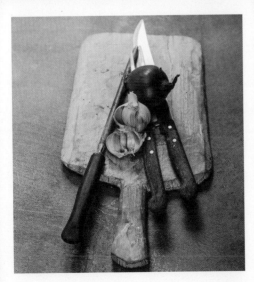

Main dishes 72

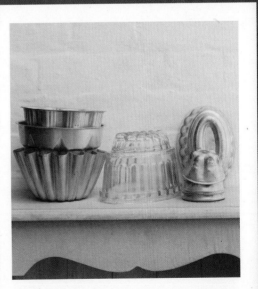

Desserts and baking 100

Index 126

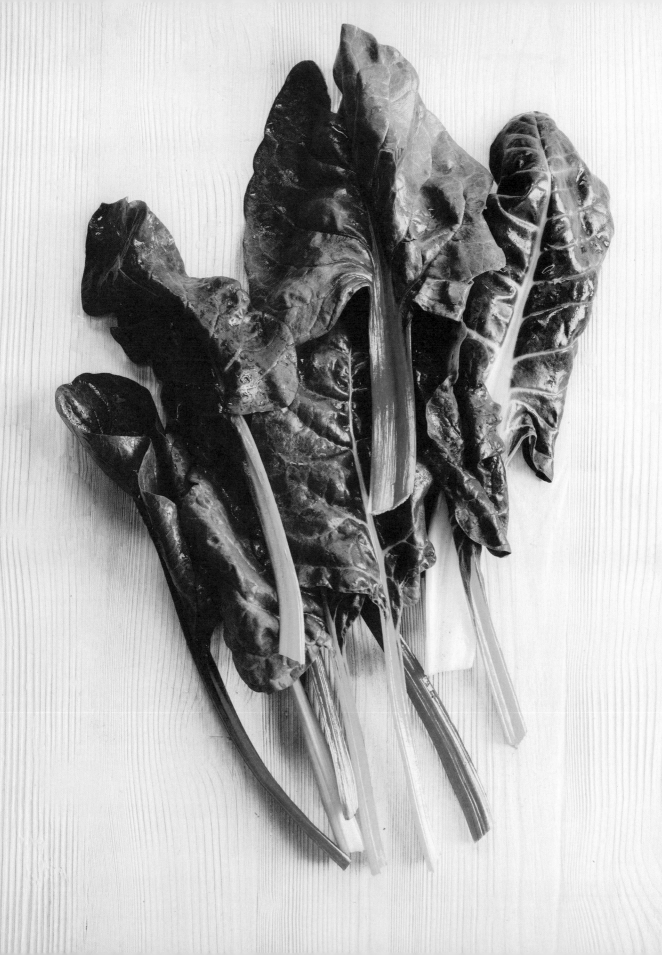

WHAT IS A SUPERFOOD?

"Superfoods" have been celebrated by nutritionists as being beneficial for health and well-being for years. These nutrient-dense ingredients offer a bundle of essential vitamins, minerals, protein, complex carbohydrates, and good monounsaturated and polyunsaturated fats. A balanced intake of these nutrients is crucial for energy, growth, repair, immunity, and essential metabolic processes. The good news doesn't stop there though—superfoods are also rich in antioxidants and phytochemicals, which can help protect us against cancers, coronary heart disease, strokes, type-2 diabetes, and obesity. No wonder we so often hear that superfoods should be top of our shopping list!

Superfoods can be bought easily from supermarkets, farmers' markets, and health-food stores and are often inexpensive. Thanks to their health-boosting qualities, they could almost be called "natural medicines," but no prescription is required and there are no negative side effects as long as they are eaten as part of a balanced diet.

The brighter the color of a fruit or vegetable, the more beneficial to health it will probably be. Choose from deep-purple blueberries; ruby-red strawberries and raspberries; bright-orange pumpkins, carrots, and mangoes; and deep-green broccoli and kale. Plant foods are packed with antioxidants and phytochemicals (biologically active plant chemicals). These help to reduce the activity of free radicals—harmful compounds produced by the body, which damage DNA and body tissues—and so they are believed to help protect the body against cancer.

Wash or scrub fruits and vegetables and eat them with the skins on where possible to boost your fiber, vitamin, and mineral intake. This is an easy way to add natural soluble fiber to your diet, which will help stave off midmorning or midafternoon munchies, and to lower cholesterol and protect against bowel cancer.

Plants aren't the only superfoods. Nuts, seeds, whole grains, oily fish, and plain yogurt with active cultures are other examples of nutrient-dense, power-packed ingredients.

When altering your diet, take small steps that you can build on instead of making major dietary changes you may struggle to maintain. There's a lot of truth in the expression "we are what we eat," and eating a range of superfoods should help you to feel fitter, lighter, and more energized, and to cope with the hustle and bustle of modern living, while improving your long-term health.

WHAT IS A HEALTHY DIET?

The key to a healthy diet is variety, so try to eat a mixture of many types of foods. Dishes offering low nutritional value, such as sugar- and fat-laden cakes and cookies, can harm you if eaten in large quantities or over a long period of time. They have been linked to obesity, type-2 diabetes, high cholesterol, heart problems, and even cancer. There is nothing wrong with the odd treat, but keep a burger and fries or a slice of chocolate cake as just that, an occasional treat.

In Western countries, 21st-century diseases are more commonly caused by dietary excess and imbalance than by nutritional deficiency. It is important to eat foods from all the main food groups: carbohydrates, proteins, fats, vitamins, and minerals. However, some foods are better than others. Opt for whole-grain carbohydrates, rich in fiber, because these take a long time to digest, leaving you feeling fuller for longer and releasing energy slowly to help you avoid mood swings and lethargy, and they are thought to help lower cholesterol.

Add sugar to foods sparingly, if at all, choosing naturally sweet fruits and dried fruits in place of highly refined white sugar.

Instead of butter and cream, choose virgin cold-pressed oils, such as olive or canola oil, or try hemp, flaxseed, or walnut oils. Low-fat versions of yogurt with active cultures, cottage cheese, cream cheese, or ricotta also make healthy options. Grill or broil meat and fish instead of frying them to lower your fat intake, and choose "clean" meats, such as protein-rich skinless turkey breast, which is low in saturated fat—the primary cause of clogged arteries. When using hard cheeses, such as cheddar, Swiss Gruyère, or Parmesan, which are high in fat, grate them so that a little goes a long way.

Cut back on sodium. Just 1 teaspoon of salt equals 2,400 milligrams of sodium. Junk food, frozen dinners, and chilled prepared meals and snacks all tend to be high in sodium.

Remember, food doesn't always need to be cooked; you can increase your intake of crisp leafy salads, fruity salsas, and fruit salads. Instead of snacking on potato chips or cookies, have an apple or a handful of dried goji berries or dates.

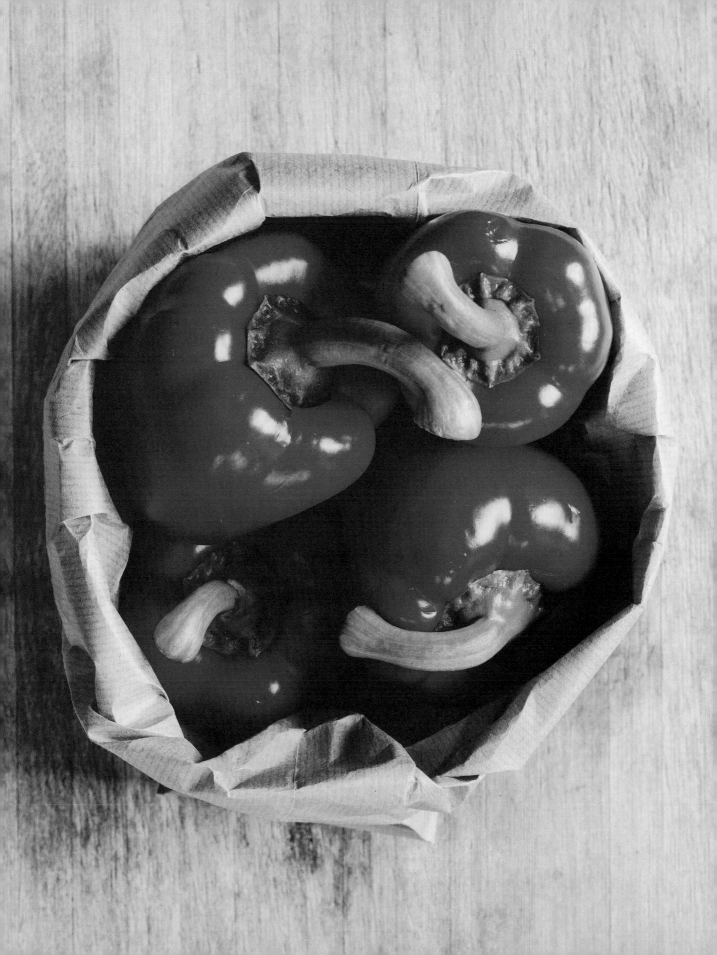

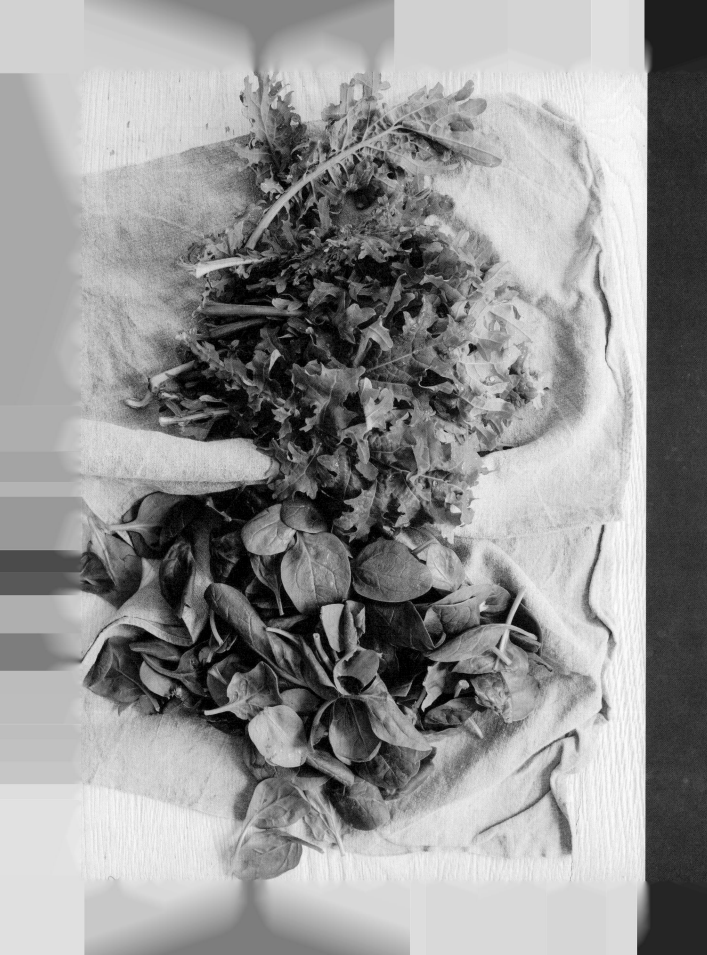

20 FABULOUS SUPERFOODS

1 Go for green: The deeper green vegetables are, the more lutein and zeaxanthin (two antioxidants related to vitamin A) they will probably contain. Broccoli, cabbage, Swiss chard, kale, arugula, spinach, and watercress are rich in chlorophyll, which assists with the oxygenation and health of blood cells, so helping to fight fatigue. They are also good sources of the B vitamins, especially folic acid, as well as immune-boosting vitamin C and vitamin K for strong bones and healthy blood clotting. Kale is a useful source of iron. Broccoli and cauliflower belong to the cabbage family and are good sources of sulfurous compounds, which may help protect against cancer.

2 Red fruit bonanza: Summery red berries, such as strawberries and raspberries, are rich in vitamin C, which aids healing and fights infection, and fiber. Cranberries help block bacterial growth, especially in the urinary tract. Their relative the blueberry is high in antioxidants, pectin to help lower cholesterol, and vitamin C. Pomegranates also contain antioxidant vitamins, as well as iron and fiber. Although high in water, red-flesh watermelons contain antioxidants, folic acid, potassium, and vitamins A and C. Pink and ruby grapefruits, along with other members of the citrus family and kiwis, are bursting with vitamin C as well as minerals and antioxidants. Packed full of antioxidants, iron, fiber, and vitamin C, dried goji berries make a great pantry standby. Tomatoes get their red color from lycopene, a carotenoid pigment that, along with the other antioxidants they contain, may help protect against free-radical damage and prostate cancer and prevent blood clots.

3 Red vegetable bonanza: Red beets get their red pigment from the antioxidants betalains, which help protect against free-radical damage and may help reduce the risk of heart disease, and they provide a wide range of vitamins, minerals, and carbohydrates. All sweet bell peppers contain vitamin C, but red bell peppers contain the most, followed by orange and yellow, then green. They are rich in antioxidants and bioflavonoids, which help neutralize free-radical damage and so are thought to help protect against cancer.

4 Sunshine fruits and vegetables: Rich in beta-carotene, this bright-orange group includes carrots, pumpkins including butternut squash, sweet potatoes, papayas, mangoes, and apricots. Beta-carotene is needed by the body to make vitamin A, an antioxidant thought to help protect against cancer and important for the integrity of each cell and to boost the immune system.

5 Autumnal apples and pears: Apples are rich in pectin (the setting agent in jellies and preserves), which helps to remove excess cholesterol and toxic metals from the digestive tract while stimulating the growth of friendly bacteria in the large intestine, boosting vitamin C, and providing a naturally sweet energy lift. Pears are healthy, too, and packed with fiber.

6　Eggs and low-fat yogurts: Eggs are packed with protein. Low-fat yogurts are a good replacement for cream as a dessert topping or base for frozen desserts, salad dressings, and marinades, and the calcium and phosphorus they contain helps boost bone strength. Probiotic yogurts, often labeled as having "active" or "live" cultures, are thought to help maintain and promote healthy bacterial balance in the digestive tract and strengthen your natural defenses, which is especially useful after taking antibiotics, which can kill good bacteria as well as bad.

7　Fabulous fish: Salmon, trout, herring, mackerel, fresh tuna, and sardines are oily fish that are rich in protein, needed for growth and the maintenance of cells. They're packed with omega-3 essential fatty acids, which help protect against heart and circulation problems and aid healthy development of the eyes and brain of a baby during pregnancy. They're a good source of minerals: selenium for growth and fertility, iodine for healthy function of the thyroid gland, vitamin B12 for the nervous system, and vitamin D for healthy bones and teeth. Try to eat one portion each week.

8　Sustaining whole grains: Avoid highly refined rice and flours. Choose brown rice for higher vitamin B levels and fiber. Opt for whole wheat or whole-grain flour for maximum fiber, or try wheat-free, gluten-free flours, such as buckwheat flour, brown rice flour, or hemp flour. Rolled oats and oatmeal make a sustaining, warming breakfast or muesli base, and taste great in cakes and baked goods. Cook barley or wheat berries in boiling water as an alternative to rice. Look for whole-grain couscous and quinoa, the only grain to contain all the essential amino acids the body requires. Rich in fiber, whole grains leave you feeling fuller for longer and help maintain a healthy digestive system, lower cholesterol, and aid good heart health.

9　Power legumes: Choose beans, either dried or canned in water, for a cheap, low-fat base to any meal. They taste great mixed with vegetables and spices, and a little added to meat or poultry makes a meal go farther. Dried legumes include cannellini beans, navy beans, chickpeas, and red kidney beans to name just a few. They all require soaking in cold water overnight and then boiling in water before use. Red lentils, which make a good base for soups; brown lentils, which are great as a salad base; or the larger green lentils, can all be used without soaking and are a good source of protein, B vitamins, and minerals. The fiber they contain helps to lower blood cholesterol, while the starch is digested and absorbed by the body slowly for a sustained energy release.

10　Nuts and seeds: Packed with protein, nuts supply many of the same minerals that meat does, such as the B vitamins, phosphorus, iron, copper, and potassium, so are good for vegetarians. They are high in fat, so add them to dishes in small amounts. Nuts are one of the richest sources of vitamin E, but this is destroyed when they are roasted, so eat raw when you can. Supermarkets now sell hemp, flaxseed, and chia seeds as well as pumpkin, sunflower, and sesame seeds. Ideally, freshly grind or chop them, so the body is able to absorb as many of the nutrients as possible. Finely ground seeds can be used in much the same way as ground almonds. Like nuts, seeds are high in calories. Flaxseed is rich in the B vitamins, magnesium, and manganese, plus omega-3 and -6 essential fatty acids. Chia seeds are also a good source of essential fatty acids as well as calcium, iron, copper, and zinc. Hemp seeds are the only seeds to contain all the essential amino acids.

11　Dates: A natural source of sweetness, dates contain fiber, potassium, manganese, magnesium, and vitamins A, B6, and K. Due to the fiber content, they're thought to help maintain a healthy colon

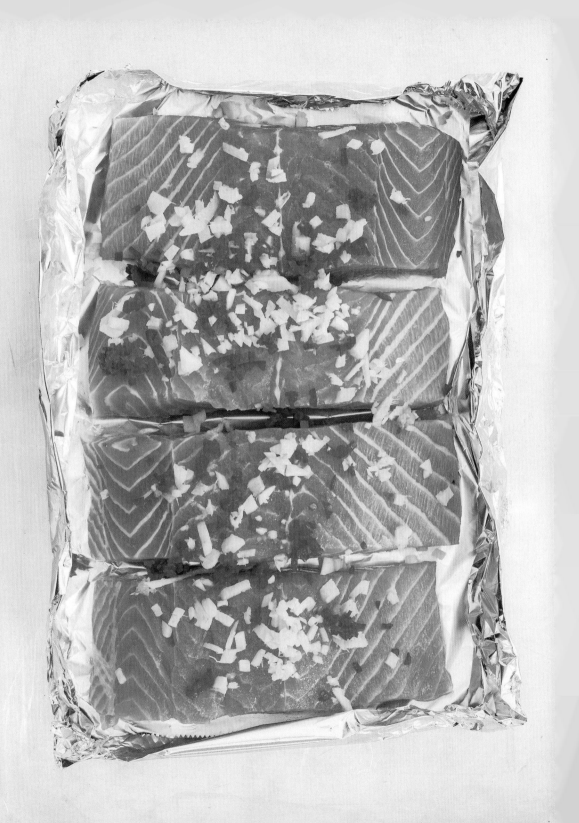

2   Secrets of soybeans: The Chinese and Japanese have long enjoyed soybeans and tofu (a soybean product). Soybeans are rich in protein, contain all the essential amino acids, vitamin E and the B vitamins, calcium, iron, and antioxidants, and are low in fat. Fiber-rich baby green soybeans, known as edamame, are sold frozen. Soy milk, made from the soaked ground beans, can be used instead of dairy milk in most recipes. Tofu is made from soybeans; dice it and add to stews, noodle dishes, or soups, or marinate in soy sauce, ginger, and garlic, then grill, dice, and add to salads or stir-fries. Soybeans help to protect against heart disease, osteoporosis, and menopausal symptoms.

3   Amazing alliums: These are members of the onion family. Garlic has been used for centuries to help fight infections, because it acts as an antimicrobial agent. Leeks are another allium with superfood properties and are noted for their concentration of the B vitamin folate, while their antioxidant and flavonoid properties mean they help protect blood vessels and blood cells.

4   Jerusalem artichokes: Packed with inulin, these knobbly roots are thought to aid beneficial bacteria in the digestive tract, while their high fiber and water content help keep our bowels healthy. They are also a good source of potassium.

5   Energizing bananas: A banana is a terrific high-energy snack and a great source of natural fruit sugars, starch, and potassium to help regulate blood pressure and lower the risk of heart attacks and strokes. It is the only fruit to contain both the amino acid tryptophan and vitamin B_6, which together produce the natural chemical serotonin, making it a good-mood food.

6   Amazing avocados: The avocado contains even more potassium than the banana. Thought to be one of the most nutritionally complete fruits, it is rich in vitamins, minerals, phytonutrients, the antioxidant lutein, and protein.

7   Seed sprouts: Think of seed sprouts as a nutritional powerhouse. As the seeds germinate and begin to sprout, their natural nutrients multiply to meet the growing needs of the young shoots. This makes them a good way to add a range of antioxidants and immune-boosting vitamins, minerals, and protein to a dish. As the seeds sprout, so the plant enzymes increase, and this aids digestion. However, children younger than five, older adults, pregnant women, and those with a weakened immune system are vulnerable to the bacteria that may be present on sprouts, so these people should not eat raw sprouts. You can purchase alfalfa sprouts from supermarkets or buy sprouting seeds and grow them from a kit following the manufacturer's directions, making sure you wash them well.

8   Turkey: High in concentrated protein, skinless and boneless turkey is low in saturated fat, total fat and sodium.

9   Semisweet chocolate: Choose semisweet chocolate that has at least 65 percent cocoa. The higher the cocoa content, the higher the flavonoids, which help to reduce infection and protect cells from damage. Semisweet chocolate also contains the mineral magnesium, needed for nerve and muscle function, and the amino acid tryptophan, which is used by the body to make serotonin.

20   Green tea: Long favored by the Chinese, green tea contains an enhanced level of antioxidants. It is thought to have antibacterial and antiviral properties. Many people believe it can help boost metabolism, aid blood pressure, and reduce bad cholesterol.

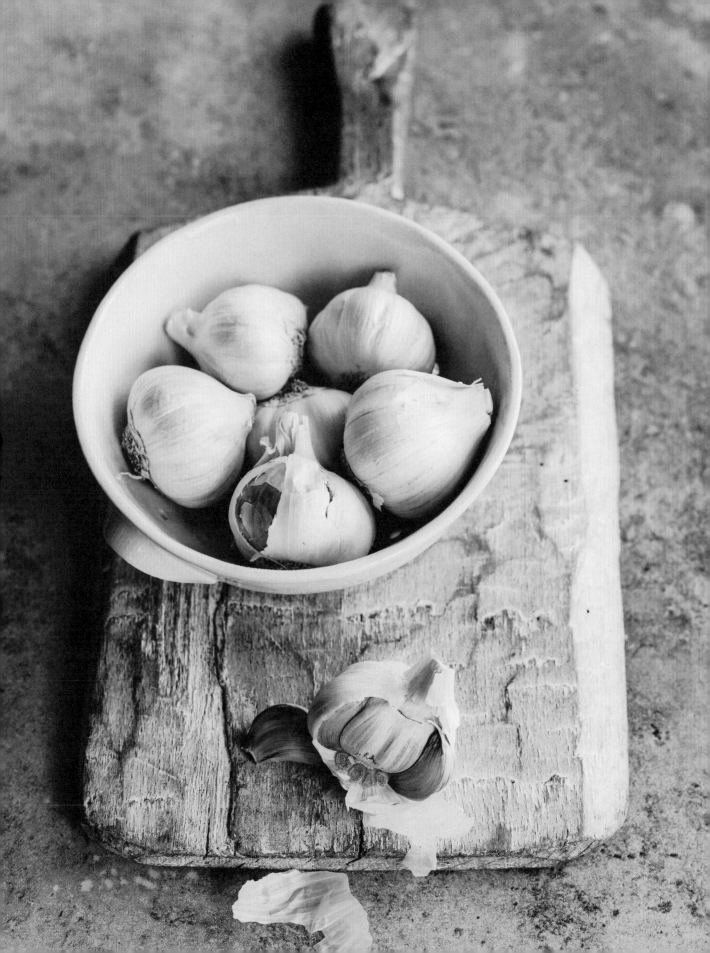

SUPER INGREDIENTS

Maca: A small, round root that was first grown in the Andes. It is thought to help fight fatigue and menopausal and menstrual discomfort and depression. It is available from health-food stores in powder form, and can be mixed into oatmeal or porridge, smoothies, or nut milks. It's a rich source of protein, minerals, vitamins C and E, and the vitamin-B group.

Spirulina: A dark-green algae, usually sold in powder form, which is rich in chlorophyll, calcium, protein, essential fatty acids, and vitamin B_{12}. Stir it into juices and smoothies.

Wheatgrass: You can buy wheatgrass as fresh grass in trays from health-food stores. Press it through a juicer, then mix it with banana or another sweet-tasting fruit, because it has a strong taste. Powdered wheatgrass is much easier to use; simply stir a teaspoon or two into smoothies, juices, or salad dressings, but be aware that it will turn everything dark green. It contains chlorophyll, vitamins A, C, and K, the vitamin-B group, iron, and potassium.

SUPERFOODS DAY BY DAY

The more superfoods you eat, the less room you will have for unhealthy foods. It doesn't take long to make a healthy stir-fry or salad. For lunch, top up sandwiches with shredded carrot or salad greens, or pack a small container of three-bean salad or coleslaw made with French dressing instead of mayonnaise, plus fresh or dried fruits.

Most fruits and vegetables are low in calories, so portion sizes can be generous. Keep a bag of apples instead of cookies or chocolate in your desk. Nuts and seeds are easy to nibble on, and are packed with protein and healthy fats, but try not to eat too many because they are also high in calories.

Changing your diet doesn't have to mean an increase in your food bill. For example, homemade soup can be quick and inexpensive to make, and extra portions can be frozen for an easy lunch. Frozen fruit, peas, green beans, corn kernels, and fish make handy standbys and can contain more vitamins and minerals than fresh ones that have sat in the refrigerator for too long.

Plan your weekly dinners and other meals; it makes shopping easier and quicker and there will be less temptation to buy junk food and processed chilled convenience meals.

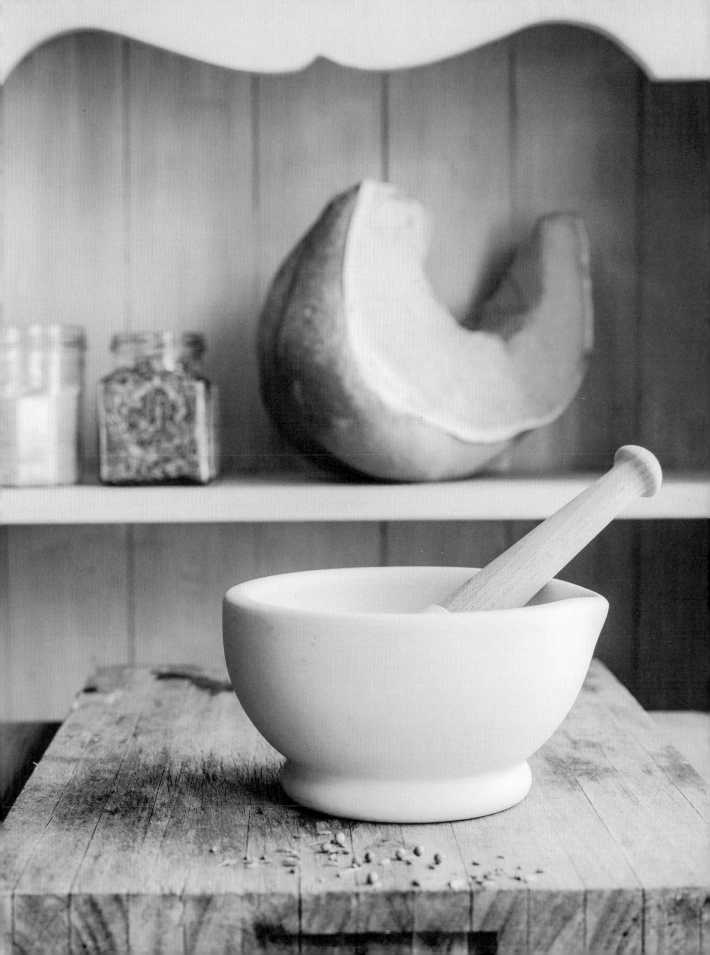

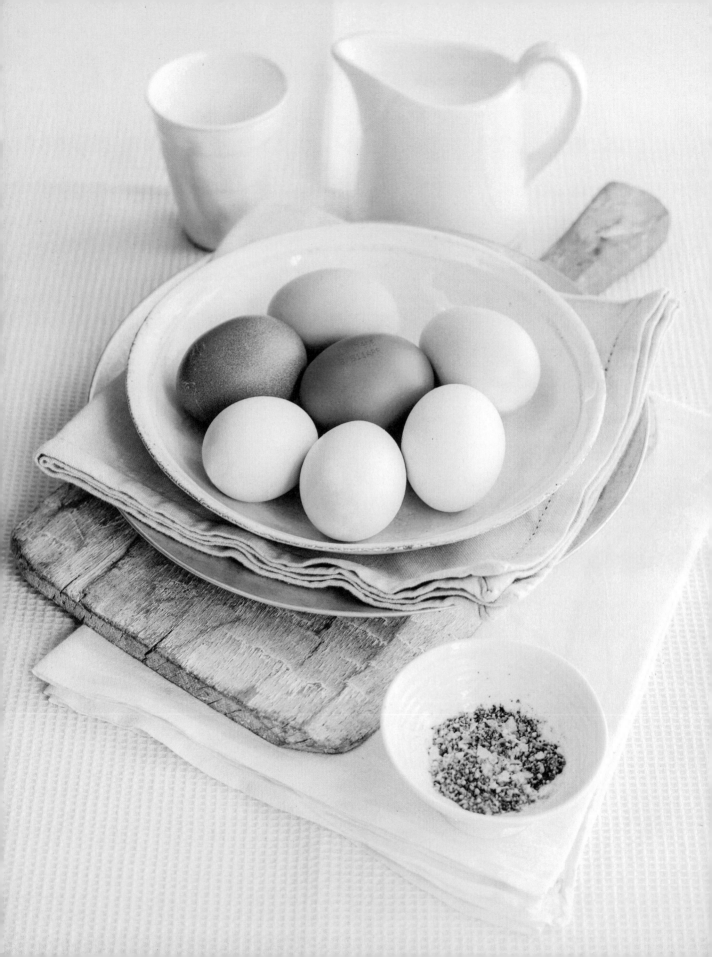

BREAKFASTS

Red beet hash 20

Eggs in red pepper and tomato sauce 22

Cinnamon pancakes with tropical fruit salad ... 24

Jumbo carrot cake cookies 26

Banana, goji, and hazelnut bread 28

Barley porridge with broiled papaya and peaches ... 30

Apple and seed muesli 33

Fruity granola cups 34

Strawberry breakfast dip 37

Yogurt with blueberries, honey, and nuts 38

Mango and kale juice 40

Avocado and fruit juice 43

RED BEET HASH

A vegetable hash is the perfect weekend brunch. This dish contains antioxidant-rich sweet potatoes, low-carbohydrate Jerusalem artichokes, and cholesterol-lowering beets.

SERVES: 4   PREP: 20 MINS   COOK: 40 MINS

12 ounces Jerusalem artichokes, unpeeled and scrubbed
5¹/2 raw beets (about 1 pound), cut into cubes
5 sweet potatoes (about 1¹/2 pounds), cut into cubes
2 tablespoons olive oil
1 red onion, coarsely chopped
2 teaspoons mild paprika
¹/2 teaspoon dry mustard
1 tablespoon fresh thyme leaves, plus extra to garnish
4 eggs
salt and pepper, to taste

1 Halve any larger artichokes. Fill the bottom of a steamer halfway with water, bring to a boil, then add the artichokes to the water. Put the beets in one half of the steamer top, cover with a lid, and steam for 10 minutes. Put the sweet potatoes in the other half of the top so the color of the beets doesn't bleed into them. Cover with a lid again and steam for an additional 10 minutes, or until all the vegetables are just tender. Drain the artichokes, peel them, and cut them into cubes.

2 Heat 1 tablespoon of oil in a large skillet over medium heat. Add the red onion and sauté for 3–4 minutes, or until beginning to soften. Add the artichokes, beets, and sweet potatoes and cook for 10 minutes, or until browned.

3 Stir in the paprika, dry mustard, and thyme and season well with salt and pepper. Make four spaces in the skillet, drizzle in the remaining oil, then crack an egg into each hole. Sprinkle the eggs with salt and pepper. Cover and cook for 4–5 minutes, or until the eggs are cooked to your liking. Spoon onto plates and serve immediately, garnished with extra thyme.

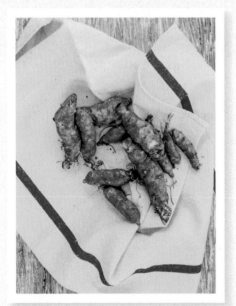

DETOX WITH ARTICHOKES

Knobbly-looking Jerusalem artichokes contain several phytonutrients, which are thought to help detoxify the liver and boost gallbladder function. They are also considered to help digestion. What's more, they're packed with fiber, helping you to feel fuller for longer.

PER SERVING: 430 CAL | 12.6G FAT | 2.7G SAT FAT | 67.4G CARBS | 25.3G SUGARS | 1.4G SALT | 11.1G FIBER | 14G PROTEIN

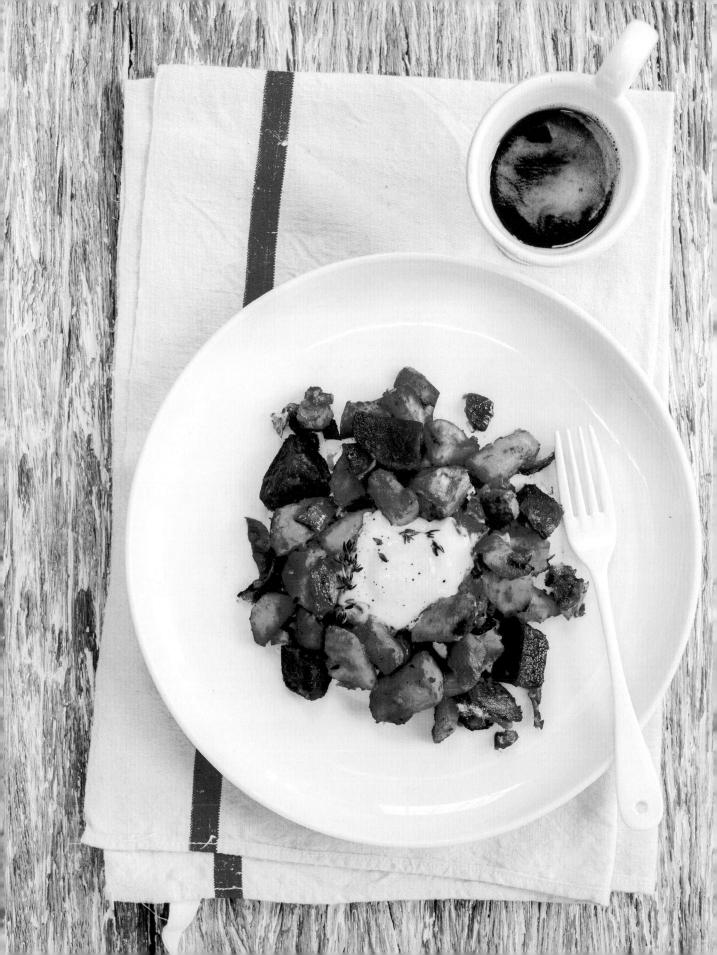

EGGS IN RED PEPPER AND TOMATO SAUCE

Protein-packed eggs are stars of the show in this simple one-pan brunch that's bursting with superfoods.

SERVES: 4 PREP: 20 MINS COOK: 30 MINS

4 large tomatoes
1¹/2 tablespoons canola oil
1 large onion, finely chopped
¹/2 teaspoon coriander seeds, crushed
¹/2 teaspoon caraway seeds, crushed
2 red bell peppers, seeded and coarsely chopped
¹/4 teaspoon crushed red pepper flakes
1 large garlic clove, thinly sliced
4 eggs
salt and pepper, to taste
1 tablespoon coarsely chopped fresh flat-leaf parsley, to garnish

1 Put the tomatoes in a shallow bowl and cover with boiling water. Let stand for 30 seconds, then drain. Slip off the skins and discard, then chop the flesh.

2 Heat the oil in a large skillet over medium heat. Add the onion, coriander seeds, and caraway seeds. Sauté, stirring occasionally, for 10 minutes, or until the onion is soft and golden.

3 Stir in the red bell peppers and red pepper flakes and sauté for an additional 5 minutes, or until softened.

4 Add the garlic and tomatoes with their seeds and juices and season with salt and pepper. Reduce the heat to low and simmer, uncovered, for 10 minutes.

5 Crack the eggs over the surface. Cover and cook for an additional 4–5 minutes, or until the eggs are cooked to your liking. Season with salt and pepper, sprinkle with the parsley, and serve immediately.

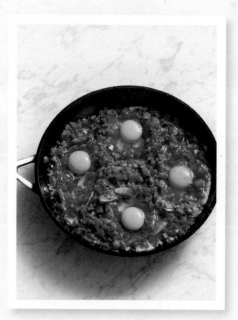

TASTY TOMATOES

Tomatoes contain vitamins A, C, and E, as well as zinc and selenium, all of which can help disarm free radicals that are produced when the body is under stress.

PER SERVING: 181 CAL | 11G FAT | 2.2G SAT FAT | 12G CARBS | 6.9G SUGARS | 0.9G SALT | 3.2G FIBER | 9G PROTEIN

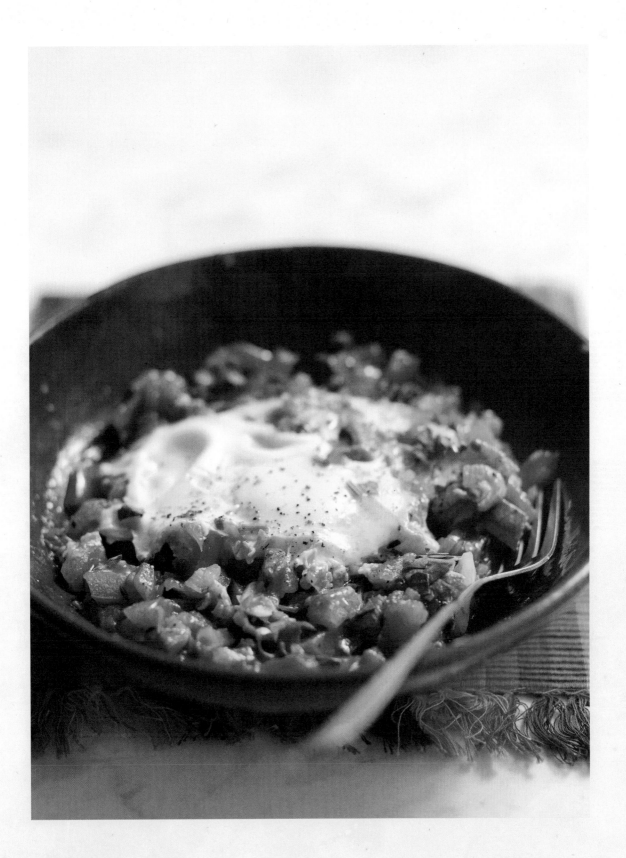

CINNAMON PANCAKES WITH TROPICAL FRUIT SALAD

Everyone loves pancakes, and these French-style crêpes, or thin pancakes, are sure to be a hit. Make the fruit salad the night before and keep it in the refrigerator to save time.

SERVES: 4   PREP: 25 MINS   COOK: 25 MINS

3/4 cup whole wheat flour
1/2 teaspoon ground cinnamon
2 eggs, beaten
1 cup unsweetened soy milk
3 tablespoons water
3 tablespoons sunflower oil

FRUIT SALAD
1 ruby grapefruit
1 1/2 cups pineapple cubes
1 cup mango cubes
finely grated zest of 1/2 lime

TO SERVE
1 1/4 cups plain soy yogurt
2 tablespoons date syrup
10 Brazil nuts, coarsely chopped (optional)

1 For the fruit salad, cut the peel and pith away from the grapefruit with a small serrated knife. Hold it above a bowl and cut between the membranes to release the segments into the bowl. Squeeze the juice from the membranes into the bowl. Add the pineapple, mango, and lime zest and mix well.

2 For the pancakes, put the flour and cinnamon in another bowl. Add the eggs, then gradually whisk in the soy milk until smooth. Whisk in the water and 1 tablespoon of oil.

3 Heat a little oil in a 7-inch skillet over medium heat, then pour out the excess oil. Pour in one-eighth of the batter, tilting the pan to swirl the batter into an even layer. Cook for 2 minutes, or until the underside is golden.

4 Loosen the pancake, then flip it over with a spatula and cook the second side for 1 minute, or until golden. Slide out of the pan and keep hot on a plate while you make another seven thin pancakes in the same way.

5 Arrange two folded pancakes on each of four plates and top with the fruit salad. Serve with a spoonful of the yogurt, drizzled with the date syrup. Top with the nuts, if using.

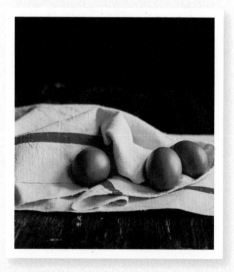

EGGSTRA SPECIAL

Eggs are loaded with protein, selenium, iron, the B vitamins, and folic acid. They contain the antioxidant lutein, too, which is believed to help protect against cataracts.

PER SERVING: 375 CAL | 14.2G FAT | 2.8G SAT FAT | 53.6G CARBS | 27.4G SUGARS | 0.2G SALT | 6.1G FIBER | 13.7G PROTEIN

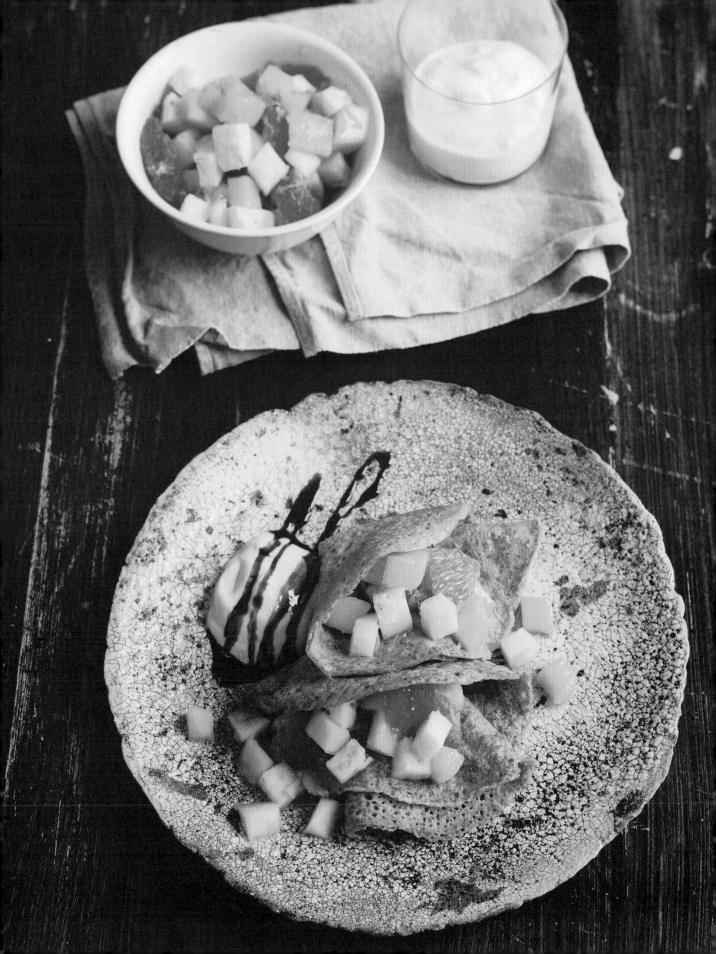

JUMBO CARROT CAKE COOKIES

These dairy-free cookies are made with coconut oil and sweetened with maple syrup, dried apricots, apple, and carrot. They're great for breakfast on the go.

MAKES: 12 COOKIES   PREP: 30 MINS   COOK: 20 MINS

2/3 cup flaxseed
2/3 cup whole wheat flour
3/4 cup rolled oats
1 teaspoon baking powder
1 teaspoon ground ginger
2 teaspoons ground cinnamon
2/3 cup finely chopped dried apricots
1 sweet, crisp apple, cored and coarsely grated
1 carrot, finely grated
1/3 cup coarsely chopped pecans
3 tablespoons coconut oil
1/2 cup maple syrup
grated zest of 1/2 orange, plus 3 tablespoons juice
1/4 cup dried coconut shavings

1   Preheat the oven to 350°F and line two baking sheets with parchment paper.

2   Put the flaxseed into a food processor or blender and process to a fine powder, then transfer to a mixing bowl. Add the flour, oats, and baking powder, followed by the ginger and cinnamon, and stir well. Add the dried apricots, apple, carrot, and pecans and stir again.

3   Warm the coconut oil in a small saucepan (or in the microwave for 30 seconds) until just liquid. Remove from the heat, then stir in the maple syrup and orange zest and juice. Pour this into the carrot mixture and stir until you have a soft dough.

4   Spoon 12 mounds of the dough onto the prepared baking sheets, then flatten them into thick 3-inch diameter circles. Sprinkle with the coconut shavings, then bake for 15–18 minutes, or until browned.

5   Serve warm or let cool, then pack into a plastic container and store in the refrigerator for up to three days.

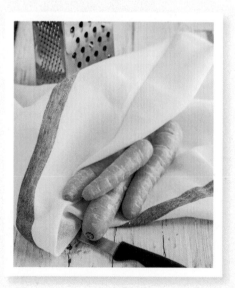

CARROTS FOR YOUR EYES

The carotenoid pigment beta-carotene that gives carrots, butternut squash, and sweet potatoes their bright-orange color is converted by the body into vitamin A, which is considered to be good for helping you to see in poor light.

PER COOKIE: 208 CAL | 10.5G FAT | 4G SAT FAT | 27G CARBS | 12.6G SUGARS | 0.3G SALT | 5.5G FIBER | 4.2G PROTEIN

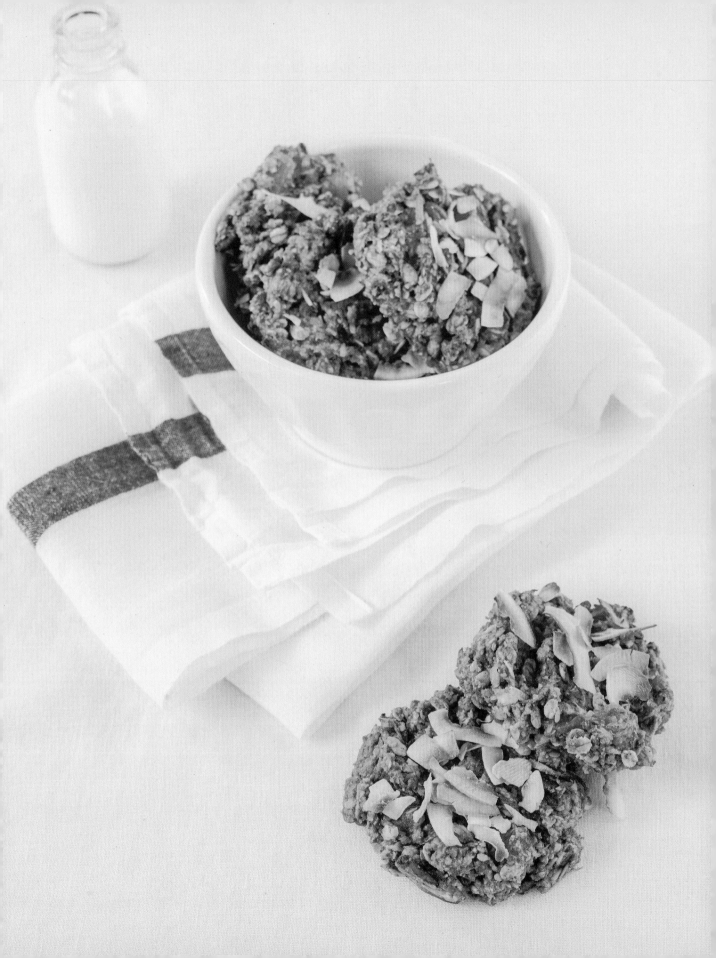

BANANA, GOJI, AND HAZELNUT BREAD

On mornings when you don't have time to eat breakfast before you leave for work, wrap a slice of this superfood-packed bread in parchment paper and eat when you get there.

MAKES: 10 SLICES
PREP: 20 MINS, PLUS COOLING   COOK: 1 HOUR

6 tablespoons butter, softened, plus extra to grease
1/2 cup firmly packed light brown sugar
2 eggs
3 bananas (about 1 pound), peeled and mashed
1 cup whole wheat flour
1 cup all-purpose flour
2 teaspoons baking powder
1/2 cup coarsely chopped unblanched hazelnuts
1/3 cup goji berries
2/3 cup dried banana chips

1 Preheat the oven to 350°F. Grease a 9 x 5 x 3-inch loaf pan and line the bottom and two long sides with a piece of parchment paper.

2 Cream the butter and sugar together in a large bowl. Beat in the eggs, one at a time, then the bananas.

3 Put the flours and baking powder into a bowl and mix well. Add to the banana mixture and beat until smooth. Add the hazelnuts and goji berries and stir well.

4 Spoon the batter into the prepared pan, smooth the top flat, then sprinkle with the banana chips. Bake for 50–60 minutes, or until the loaf is well risen, has cracked slightly, and a toothpick inserted into the center comes out clean.

5 Let cool for 5 minutes, then loosen the edges with a blunt knife and turn out onto a wire rack. Let cool completely, then peel away the paper. Store in an airtight container for up to three days.

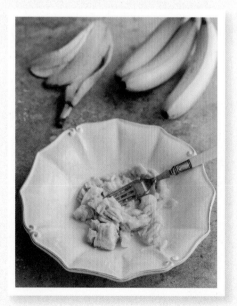

HIGH-ENERGY BANANAS

Naturally rich in fruit sugar and starch, bananas are a great energy-boosting food. They contain plenty of potassium, which can help to regulate blood pressure and lower the risk of heart attacks and strokes. They also contain the amino acid tryptophan and vitamin B_6, which together help in the production of mood-boosting serotonin.

PER SLICE: 276 CAL | 10G FAT | 2.5G SAT FAT | 43G CARBS | 19G SUGARS | 0.8G SALT | 3.5G FIBER | 5.5G PROTEIN

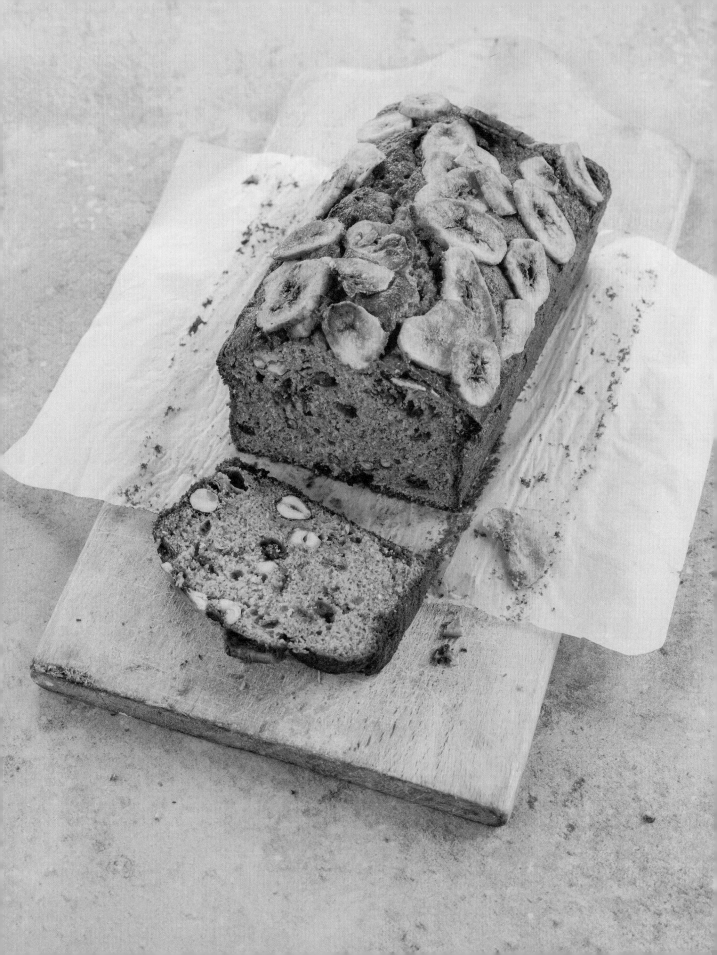

BARLEY PORRIDGE WITH BROILED PAPAYA AND PEACHES

Forget about thick, stodgy oatmeal—this healthier, lighter, dairy-free porridge is made with high-fiber barley flakes for an energizing start to the day.

SERVES: 4   PREP: 10 MINS   COOK: 10 MINS

2 cups barley flakes
1 cup rolled oats
1½ cups cold water
3 cups unsweetened almond milk
4 teaspoons maca (see page 16)
2 peaches, halved, pitted, and sliced
1 papaya, halved, seeded, peeled, and sliced
4 teaspoons honey, plus extra to serve
½ teaspoon ground cinnamon

1 Put the barley flakes, rolled oats, water, and almond milk into a saucepan. Bring to a boil over medium–high heat, then reduce the heat to medium and simmer for 5–10 minutes, stirring often, until soft and thickened. Stir in the maca.

2 Meanwhile, preheat the broiler to medium–high. Line the broiler rack with aluminum foil, then lay the peaches and papaya on top, drizzle with the honey, and sprinkle with the cinnamon. Broil for 3–4 minutes, or until hot and just beginning to caramelize.

3 Spoon the porridge into bowls, top with the hot peaches and papaya, and drizzle with a little extra honey, if desired.

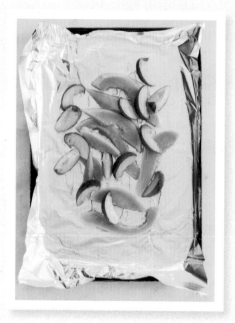

POWER PAPAYA

The beautiful, orangey-yellow tropical papaya is bursting with vitamin C, potassium, and folic acid. It also contains vitamins A and E, two antioxidants that are thought to protect against heart disease and colon cancer. Papayas are believed to be good for the skin, protecting against wrinkles, and for the eyes.

PER SERVING: 291 CAL | 4.3G FAT | 0.5G SAT FAT | 58G CARBS | 25.3G SUGARS | 0.2G SALT | 8.5G FIBER | 8.3G PROTEIN

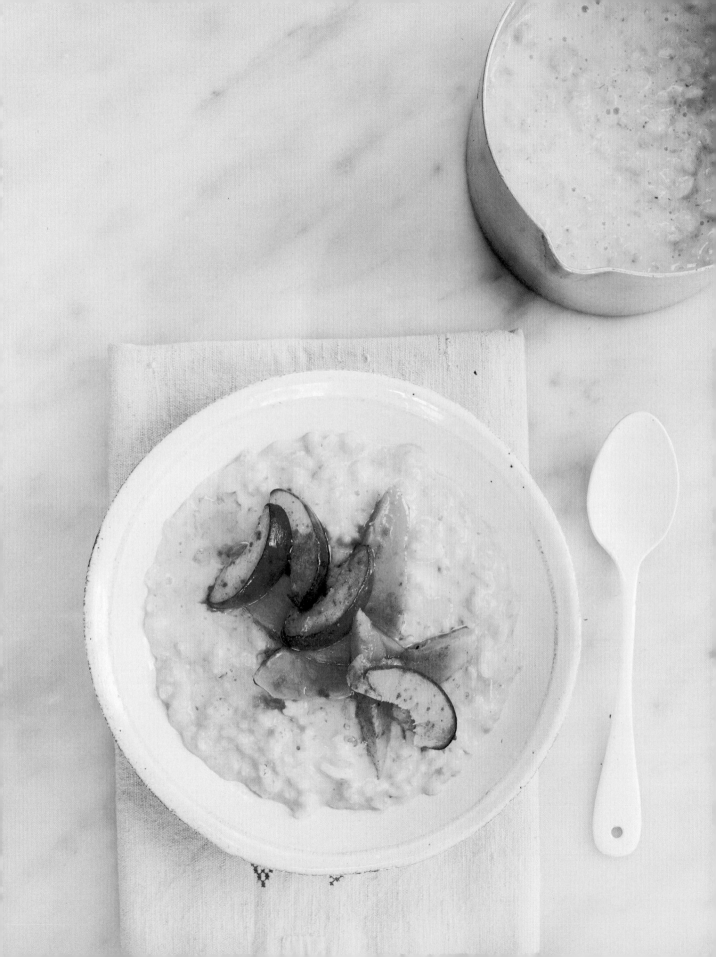

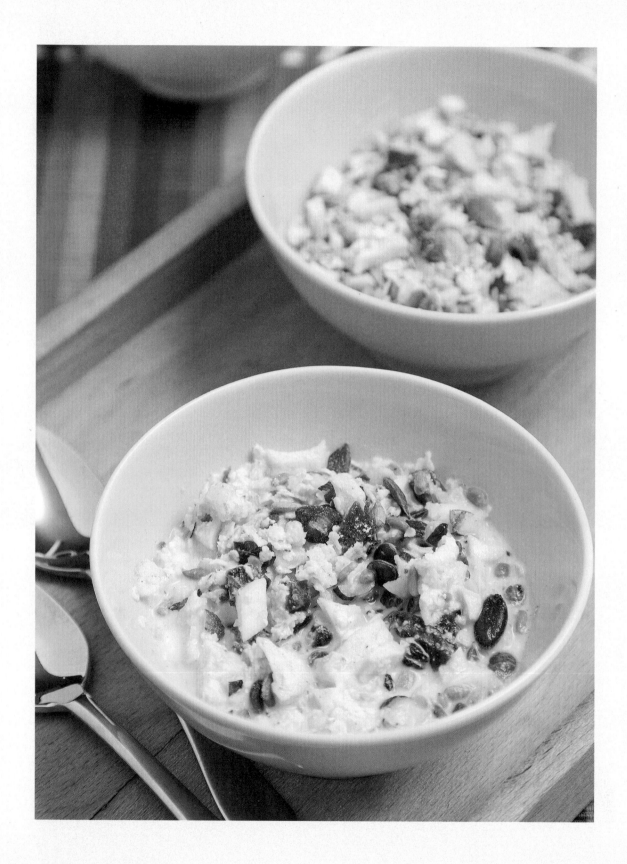

APPLE AND SEED MUESLI

Nutty and fruity, this is a delicious and healthy start to the day.
Serve it with milk or yogurt.

SERVES: 10
PREP: 15 MINS, PLUS COOLING   COOK: 4 MINS

1/2 cup sunflower seeds
1/3 cup pumpkin seeds
3/4 cup coarsely chopped hazelnuts
2 3/4 cups buckwheat flakes
2 1/2 cups rice flakes
1 1/4 cups millet flakes
1 1/3 cups coarsely chopped dried apple
3/4 cup coarsely chopped dried dates

1   Put a skillet over medium heat. Add the sunflower seeds, pumpkin seeds, and hazelnuts and toast, shaking the pan frequently, for 4 minutes, or until golden brown. Transfer to a large bowl and let cool.

2   Add the buckwheat flakes, rice flakes, millet flakes, dried apple, and dates to the bowl and mix well. Store in an airtight container for up to five days.

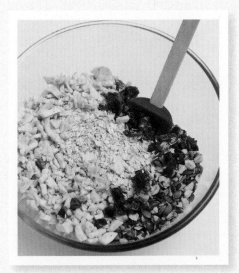

BEAUTIFUL BUCKWHEAT

Buckwheat is a seed, although many people mistakenly think of it as a grain. It is a nutrition powerhouse, containing plenty of protein. Because of its amino acid content, it can boost the protein content of beans and grains eaten on the same day. It is also a good source of fiber.

PER SERVING: 319 CAL | 13G FAT | 1.4G SAT FAT | 47.9G CARBS | 15.5G SUGARS | TRACE SALT | 5.6G FIBER | 8.9G PROTEIN

FRUITY GRANOLA CUPS

Granola is easy to make, and a wonderful standby ingredient—
just add yogurt and fruit when you're ready for breakfast.

SERVES: 6   PREP: 25 MINS   COOK: 35 MINS

1/4 cup steel-cut oats
1 cup rolled oats
1/2 cup coarsely chopped unblanched almonds
2 tablespoons pumpkin seeds
2 tablespoons sunflower seeds
2 tablespoons flaxseed, coarsely ground
1/2 teaspoon ground cinnamon
3 tablespoons maple syrup
1 tablespoon olive oil
1/4 cup dried goji berries

TO SERVE (SERVES 2)
1 cup granola
juice of 1 orange
1/2 cup Greek-style plain yogurt
1 crisp, sweet apple, cored, and coarsely grated
2/3 cup hulled and sliced strawberries
1/3 cup blueberries

1   Preheat the oven to 325°F. Put the steel-cut oats, rolled oats, and almonds in a bowl. Stir in the pumpkin seeds, sunflower seeds, and flaxseed, then the cinnamon, maple syrup, and oil.

2   Transfer the granola to a roasting pan, then spread into an even layer. Bake for 30–35 minutes, or until golden brown all over, stirring every 5–10 minutes and mixing any browner granola from the edges of the pan into the center after 15 minutes.

3   Stir in the goji berries, then let cool. Pack into an airtight container and store in the refrigerator for up to five days.

4   When ready to serve, spoon a scant 1/2 cup granola into each of two glasses or bowls, keeping a little back for the top. Moisten with the orange juice. Mix the yogurt with the apple and spoon it over the granola, then top with the strawberries and blueberries and sprinkle with the remaining granola.

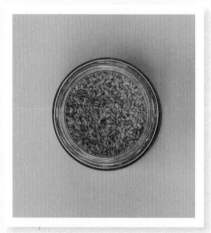

PROTECTIVE FLAXSEED

Grinding flaxseed in a food processor, blender, or spice mill means you can use them in cooking in the same way as ground almonds (almond meal). It also means they are in a form that the body can process more easily, so that larger amounts of the essential omega-3 fatty acids, needed for heart health can be absorbed. They are rich in lignans, antioxidants that help protect the body against cancer, and in the B vitamins, minerals, and fiber.

PER SERVING: 402 CAL | 13.4G FAT | 1.6G SAT FAT | 57.6G CARBS | 28.7G SUGARS | TRACE SALT | 9.3G FIBER | 15G PROTEIN

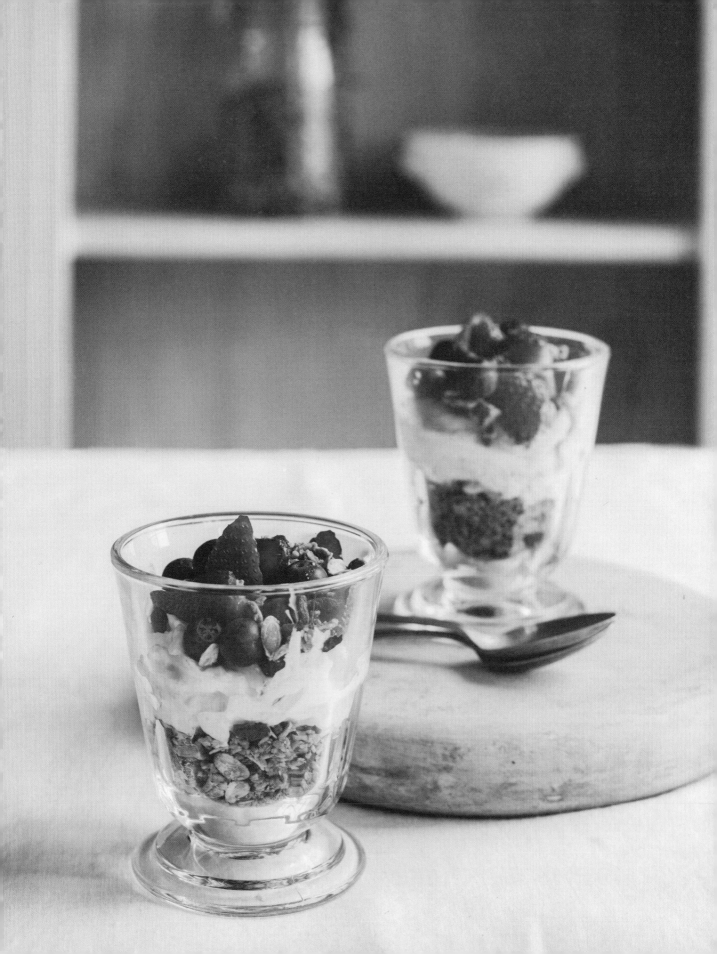

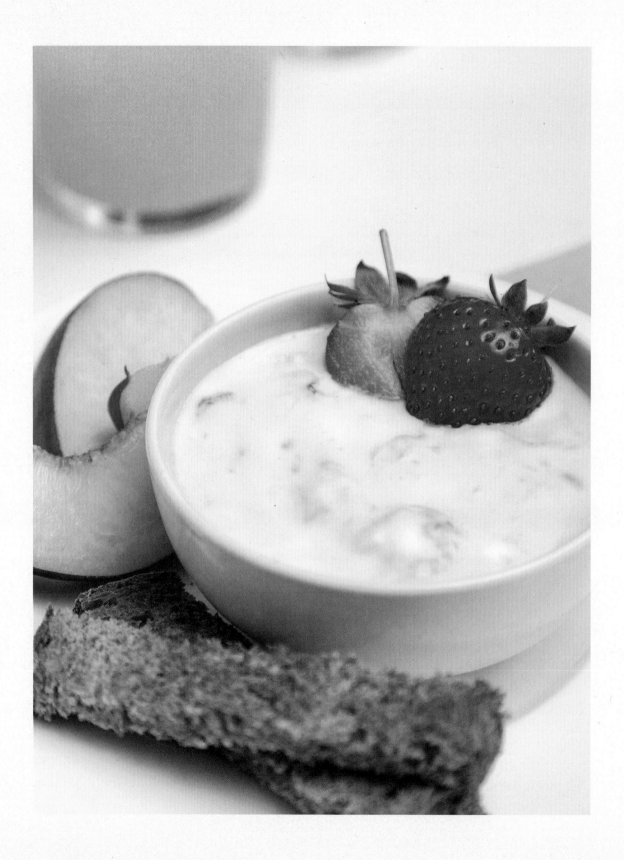

STRAWBERRY BREAKFAST DIP

This light and summery breakfast is rich in calcium, vitamin C, and antioxidants, and it can be prepared in advance and stored in the refrigerator.

SERVES: 4   PREP: 10 MINS   COOK: 5 MINS

2/3 cup hulled and coarsely chopped strawberries, plus extra, halved, to decorate
1 cup plain fromage blanc, quark, or Greek-style yogurt
1 teaspoon lemon juice
4 slices of whole-grain bread
2 nectarines, halved, pitted, and cut into wedges

1   Put the strawberries in a blender and process to a puree, then pour into a mixing bowl. Stir in the fromage blanc and lemon juice. Cover and chill in the refrigerator if you have time.

2   Toast the bread and cut it into strips. Spoon the strawberry mixture into four bowls and place each on a plate. Arrange the nectarine wedges and toast strips on the plates to use as dippers. Decorate the dip with halves of strawberries and serve immediately.

STRAWBERRY SUNSHINE

Natural sugars found in the strawberries and nectarines in this breakfast are absorbed by the body more slowly than those from a high-energy drink. Strawberries are an excellent source of vitamin C, manganese, and fiber.

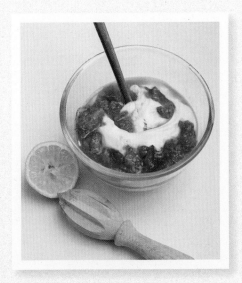

PER SERVING: 166 CAL | 5G FAT | 3G SAT FAT | 24G CARBS | 13G SUGARS | 0.4G SALT | 4G FIBER | 6.5G PROTEIN

YOGURT WITH BLUEBERRIES, HONEY, AND NUTS

Greek-style yogurt topped with fresh berries, honey, and nuts is quick to make and a delicious breakfast treat.

SERVES: 4
PREP: 10 MINS, PLUS CHILLING   COOK: 5 MINS

3 tablespoons honey
1/2 cup mixed unsalted nuts
1/2 cup Greek-style plain yogurt
1 1/3 cups blueberries

1   Heat the honey in a small saucepan over medium heat. Stir in the nuts until well coated. Remove from the heat and let cool slightly.

2   Spoon the yogurt into four bowls, then spoon the nuts and blueberries over the yogurt. Serve immediately.

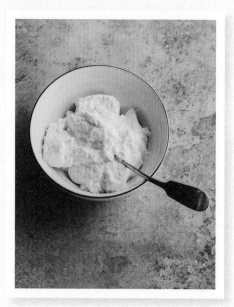

SAY YES TO YOGURT

Yogurt is an excellent source of calcium. It is also packed with high-quality protein, magnesium, and a variety of vitamins. Yogurt with live or active bacteria known as probiotics has extra benefits; these live in your digestive tract and help in the fight against infection.

PER SERVING: 237 CAL | 12.9G FAT | 2.7G SAT FAT | 27G CARBS | 19.3G SUGARS | TRACE SALT | 3.1G FIBER | 7.3G PROTEIN

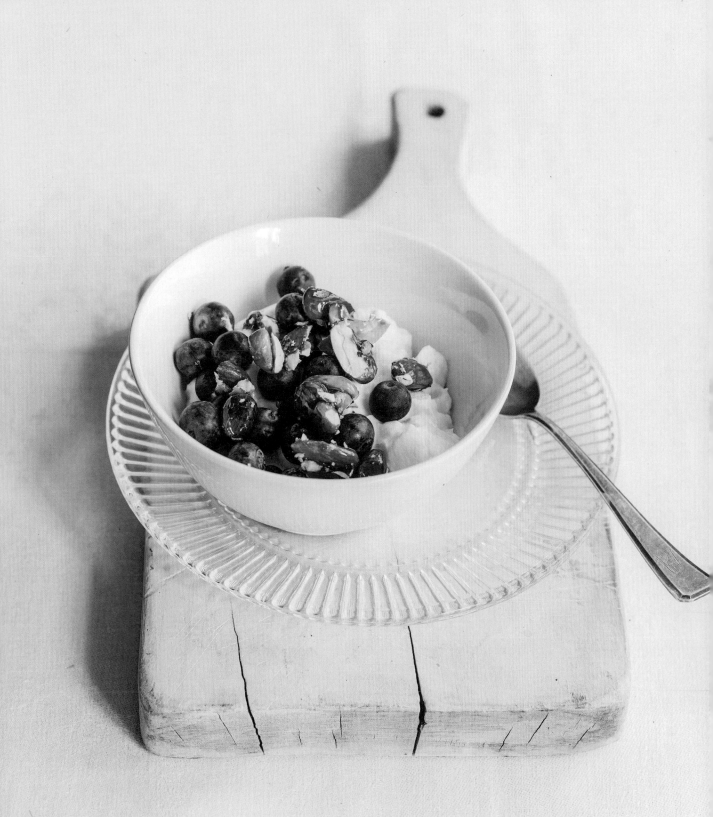

MANGO AND KALE JUICE

Mango's natural sweetness balances the kale in this health-boosting juice, and its perfumed flavor makes it refreshing as well as delicious.

SERVES: 1   PREP: 10 MINS

1 tablespoon sesame seeds
juice of 1/2 lime
1/2 cup torn green curly kale pieces
1 mango, pitted, peeled, and coarsely chopped
1 cup unsweetened rice, almond, or soy milk
small handful of crushed ice

1 Put the sesame seeds into a food processor or blender and process to a fine powder. Add the lime juice, kale, and mango and process until blended.

2 Add the milk and crushed ice and process again, until smooth. Pour into a glass and serve immediately.

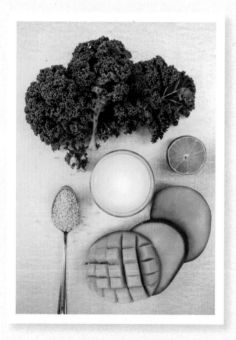

KALE KICK-START

Kale has loads of calcium, vitamin C, B vitamins, and beta-carotene. The antioxidant lutein helps protect the eyes against macular degeneration, while indoles offer protection against estrogen-related cancers, and sulforaphane may help boost the liver's ability to detox carcinogenic compounds.

PER SERVING: 347 CAL | 9.9G FAT | 1.5G SAT FAT | 57.7G CARBS | 46.4G SUGARS | 0.1G SALT | 8.5G FIBER | 12.9G PROTEIN

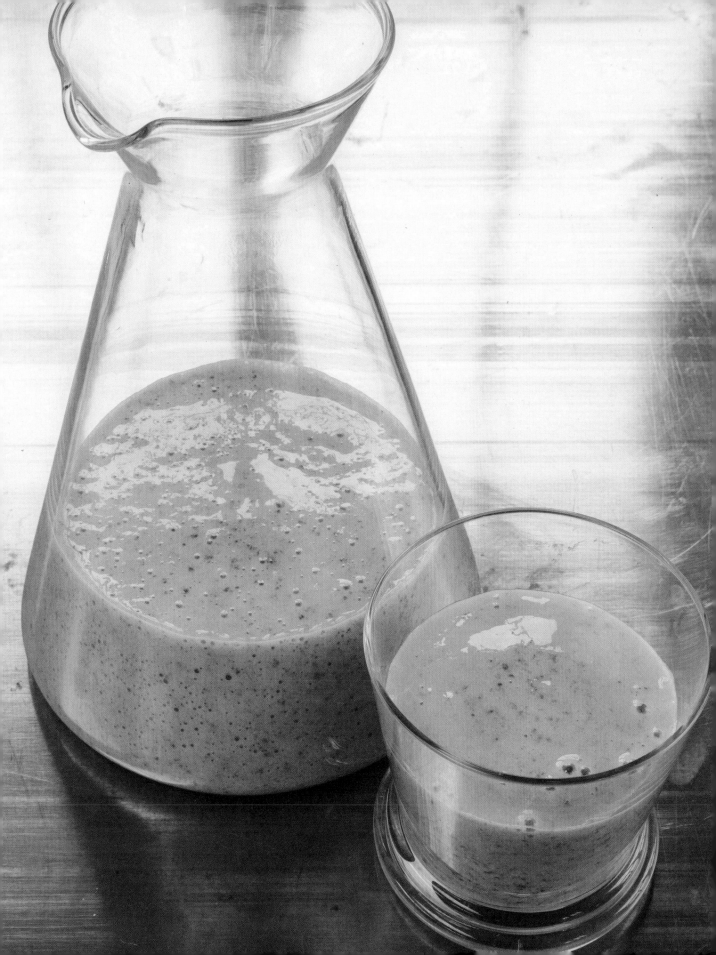

AVOCADO AND FRUIT JUICE

Protect your body from the inside out with this fresh, fruity drink that is bursting with antioxidants.

SERVES: 1 PREP: 10 MINS

1/2 avocado, pitted, peeled, and coarsely chopped
3/4 cup blueberries
3/4 cup hulled strawberries
juice of 1 tangerine or small orange
1/2 cup cold water
small handful of crushed ice (optional)

1 Put the avocado, blueberries, strawberries, tangerine juice, and water into a food processor or blender and process until blended.

2 Add the crushed ice, if using, and process again until smooth. Pour into a glass and serve.

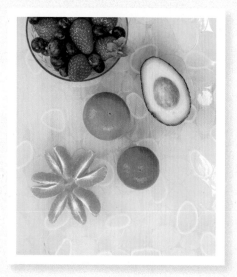

GOOD·FOR·YOU ORANGES

Oranges contain high concentrations of vitamin C, vitamin A, antioxidants, flavonoids, potassium, calcium, magnesium, and fiber. They are also thought to help prevent some cancers.

PER SERVING: 250 CAL | 15G FAT | 3.5G SAT FAT | 18G CARBS | 18G SUGARS | TRACE SALT | 6G FIBER | 3G PROTEIN

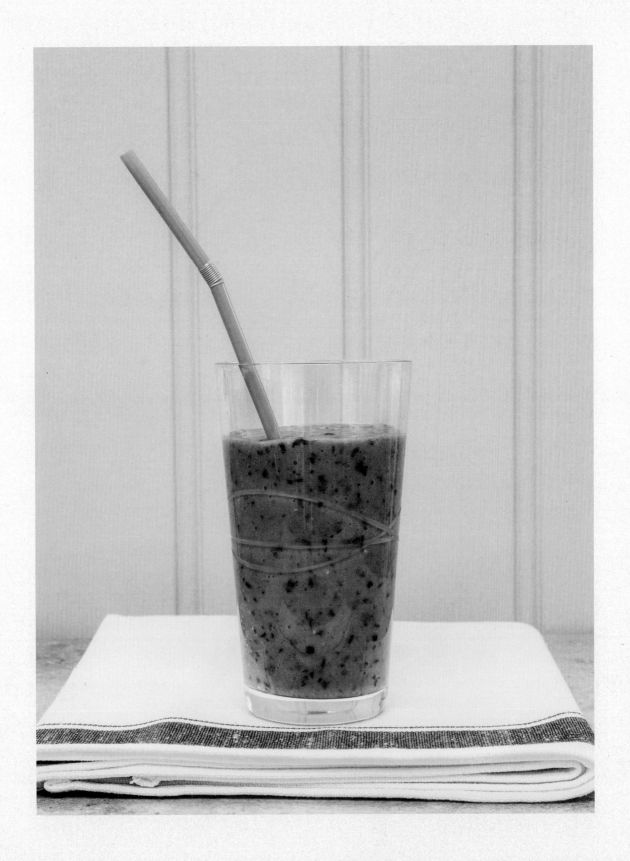

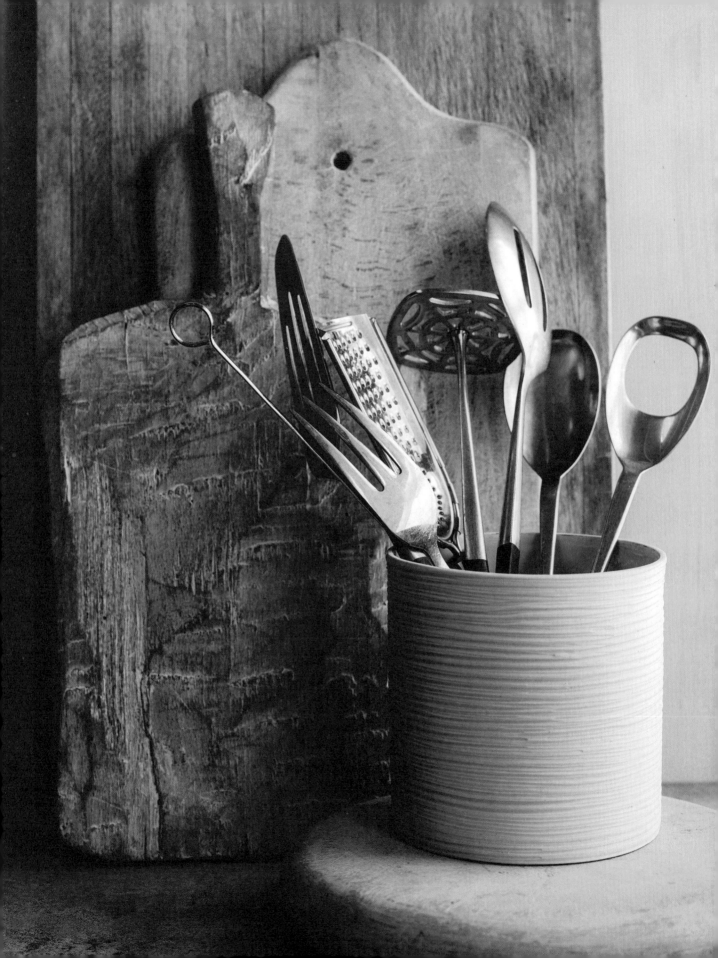

LUNCHES AND SNACKS

Ceviche   46

Lentil and spinach soup   48

Sweet red pepper and tomato soup   50

Shrimp-filled baked sweet potatoes   52

Quinoa salad with fennel and orange   54

Vietnamese tofu and noodle salad   56

Roasted beet and squash salad   58

Supergreen salad   60

Cranberry and red cabbage coleslaw   62

Sweet potato fries   64

Guacamole dip   67

Power balls   68

Honey and blueberry bars   71

CEVICHE

Tangy and tongue-tinglingly good! The fish must be superfresh for this Mexican favorite, which is bursting with chile and sweet-and-sour flavors.

SERVES: 4   PREP: 30 MINS   CHILL: 1¹/₂ HOURS

2 ruby grapefruits
7 ounces sea bass fillets, skinned, pin-boned, and cut into cubes
10¹/₂ ounces trout fillets, skinned, pin-boned, and cut into cubes
finely grated zest and juice of 2 limes
1 red chile, seeded and finely chopped
¹/₂ red onion, finely chopped
1 tablespoon virgin olive oil
¹/₃ cup finely chopped fresh cilantro
2¹/₄ cups mixed baby spinach, watercress, and arugula salad
salt and pepper, to taste

1   Cut the peel and pith away from the grapefruits with a small serrated knife. Hold each one above a bowl and cut between the membranes to release the segments into the bowl. Squeeze the juice from the membranes into the bowl.

2   Put the sea bass and trout into a ceramic or glass bowl, sprinkle with the lime zest and juice and chile, then add the red onion, grapefruit segments and juice, and oil. Season well with salt and pepper, then gently stir so all the fish is evenly coated in the lime juice.

3   Cover and chill in the refrigerator for 1–1¹/₂ hours, or until the fish has taken on a cooked appearance, with the sea bass bright white and the trout a paler, even pink.

4   Add the cilantro and stir gently. Arrange the mixed green salad on four plates and spoon the ceviche on top, then serve immediately.

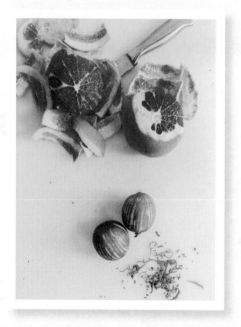

COOL CITRUS

Citrus fruits, such as limes, oranges, and grapefruits, are bursting with vitamin C. This is a highly unstable vitamin, which is destroyed by heat, so try to eat them raw. It is needed daily for healthy gums and teeth, healing wounds, and the production of collagen. Eating vitamin C-rich fruits with iron-rich spinach, watercress, and arugula enables the body to absorb more of the iron.

PER SERVING: 209 CAL | 7.8G FAT | 1.3G SAT FAT | 13.5G CARBS | 10.8G SUGARS | 0.9G SALT | 2.2G FIBER | 21.2G PROTEIN

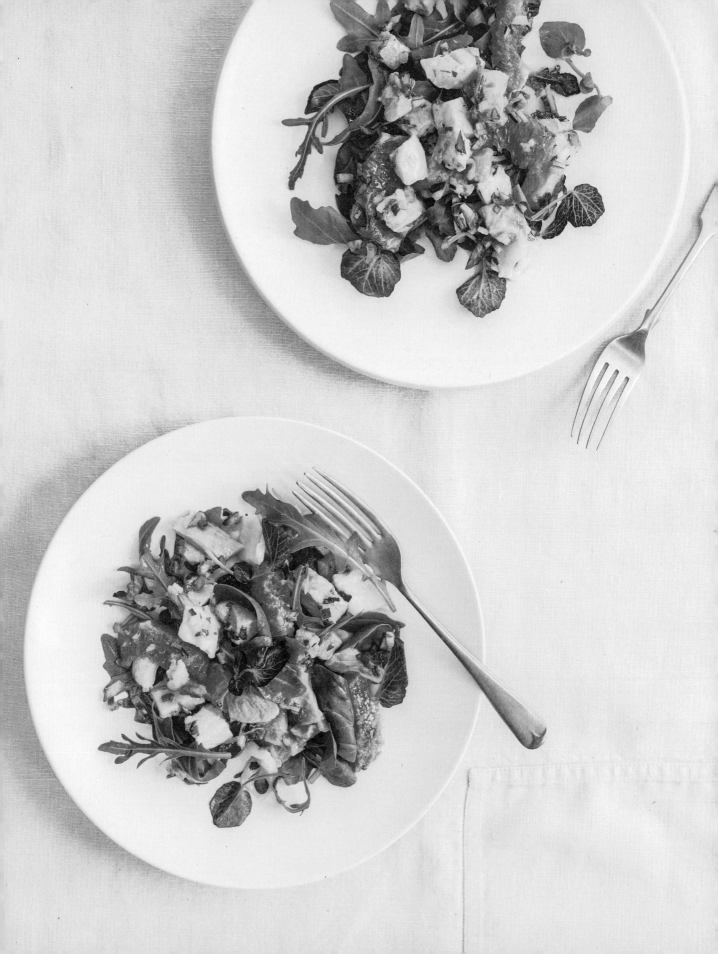

LENTIL AND SPINACH SOUP

A beautifully fresh, light, and fragrant soup that's easy to make and packed with nutrients.

SERVES: 4   PREP: 15 MINS   COOK: 45 MINS

1 teaspoon vegetable oil
1 onion, finely chopped
2 garlic cloves, finely chopped
2 celery stalks, finely chopped
3 carrots, finely chopped
1/2 teaspoon chili powder
1 teaspoon smoked paprika
1 teaspoon cumin seeds
1 cup dried red lentils, washed
4 cups vegetable stock
1 cup coarsely chopped spinach
6 cherry tomatoes, halved
salt and pepper, to taste
1/4 cup plain yogurt, to serve (optional)
4 pita breads, cut into slices, to serve (optional)

1   Heat the oil in a large saucepan over medium heat. Add the onion, garlic, celery, and carrots and cook for 4–5 minutes, or until starting to soften.

2   Add the chili powder, paprika, and cumin seeds and cook for 1 minute, stirring constantly.

3   Add the red lentils and stock, then season with salt and pepper. Bring to a boil, then cook for 10 minutes. Cover and reduce the heat to low, then simmer gently for an additional 20–25 minutes, or until the vegetables and lentils are cooked.

4   Add the spinach and tomatoes and cook for 5 minutes, or until the spinach has wilted. Taste and season again, if needed. Serve in four bowls, with a tablespoon of yogurt in each bowl and the pita breads, if using.

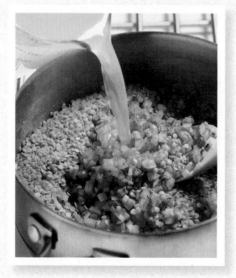

LOVELY LENTILS

Lentils are a good source of protein and are rich in fiber. It is thought they can help reduce bad cholesterol and stabilize blood-sugar levels, slowing down the rate at which sugar is absorbed by the body.

PER SERVING: 255 CAL | 4.3G FAT | 1.5G SAT FAT | 43.1G CARBS | 7.9G SUGARS | 3.3G SALT | 8.9G FIBER | 15.3G PROTEIN

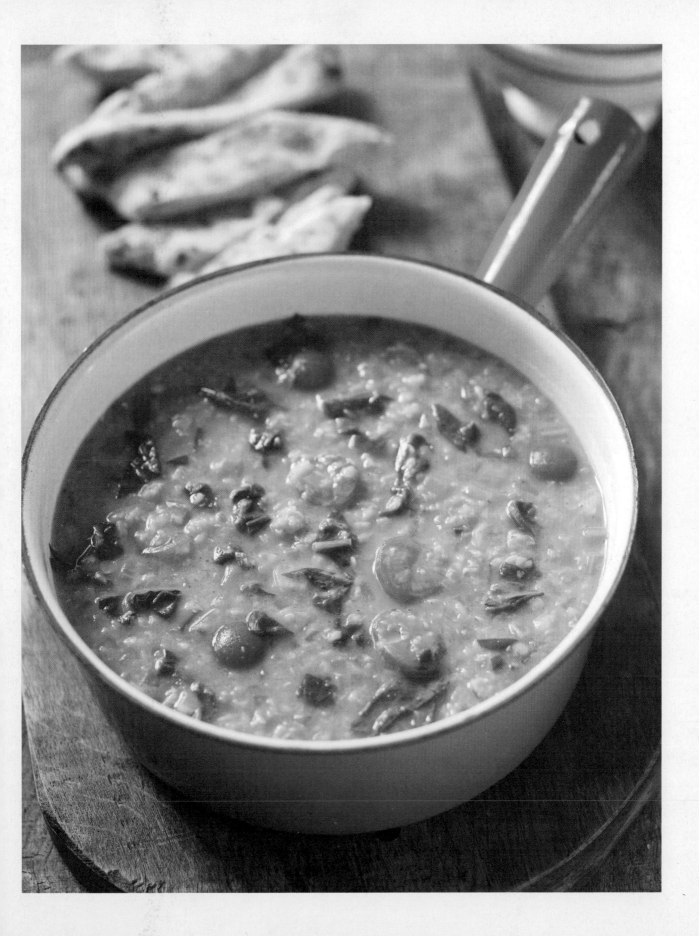

SWEET RED PEPPER AND TOMATO SOUP

This warming and comforting soup is brimming with health-boosting, antioxidant-rich vegetables.

SERVES: 4   PREP: 10 MINS   COOK: 35 MINS

1 tablespoon olive oil
2 tablespoons cold water
2 red bell peppers, seeded and finely chopped
1 garlic clove, finely chopped
1 onion, finely chopped
1 (14 1/2-ounce) can diced tomatoes
5 cups vegetable stock
salt and pepper, to taste
fresh basil leaves, to garnish

1 Put the oil, water, red bell peppers, garlic, and onion in a saucepan over medium–low heat and cook for 5–10 minutes, or until all the vegetables have softened. Cover and simmer for 10 minutes.

2 Add the tomatoes and stock and season with salt and pepper. Simmer, uncovered, for 15 minutes. Serve garnished with basil leaves.

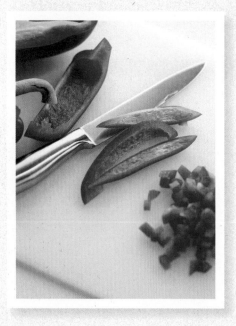

RED PEPPER BOOST

All sweet bell peppers are rich in vitamins A, C, and K, but red peppers are simply bursting with them. Antioxidant vitamins A and C help to prevent cell damage, cancer, and diseases related to aging, and they support immune function. They also reduce inflammation, such as that found in arthritis and asthma.

PER SERVING: 97 CAL | 5.4G FAT | 1.7G SAT FAT | 12.8G CARBS | 7.1G SUGARS | 3.6G SALT | 3.2G FIBER | 2.2G PROTEIN

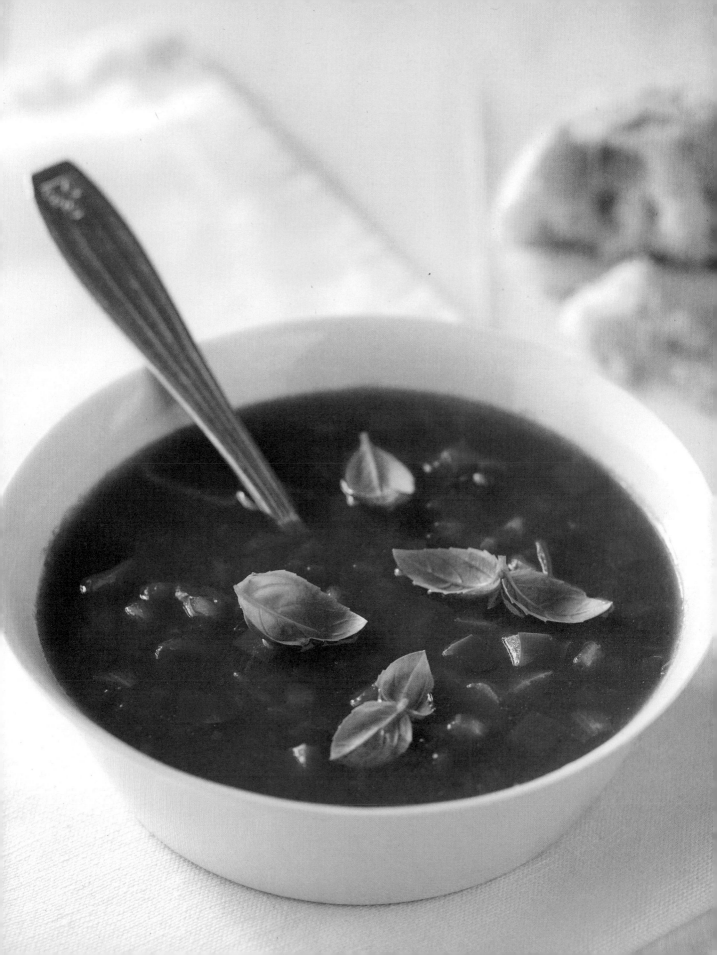

SHRIMP-FILLED BAKED SWEET POTATOES

We all love baked potatoes, and this healthy lunch is topped with low-fat cottage cheese, an antioxidant-boosting mango and corn salsa, and protein-powered shrimp.

SERVES: 4   PREP: 5 MINS   COOK: 1 HOUR

4 small sweet potatoes, scrubbed and pricked with a fork
1/2 cup frozen corn kernels
2 plum tomatoes, cut into cubes
4 scallions, finely chopped
1 mango, pitted, peeled, and cut into cubes
1/3 cup finely chopped fresh cilantro
1 red chile, seeded and finely chopped (optional)
10 1/2 ounces cooked and peeled shrimp
finely grated zest and juice of 1 lime
1 1/4 cups low-fat cottage cheese
salt and pepper, to taste

1 Preheat the oven to 400°F. Put the sweet potatoes on a baking sheet and bake for 1 hour, or until they feel soft when gently squeezed.

2 Meanwhile, bring a saucepan of water to a boil, add the frozen corn kernels, and cook for 3 minutes, or until tender. Drain into a strainer, then rinse under cold running water.

3 Put the tomatoes, scallions, and mango in a bowl, then stir in the cilantro, red chile, if using, and corn kernels and season with salt and pepper. Cover and chill in the refrigerator.

4 Put the shrimp and lime zest and juice in another bowl and season with salt and pepper. Cover and chill in the refrigerator.

5 Put the sweet potatoes on a serving plate, slit them in half, then open them out. Top with spoonfuls of the cottage cheese, then fill with the salsa and shrimp.

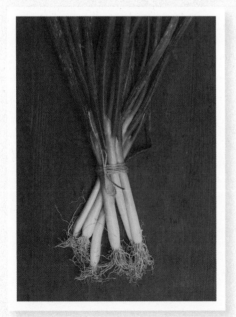

SUPER SCALLIONS

Scallions are small, immature plants of the onion family. Because they are leafy greens, they contain more plant-derived antioxidants and fiber than onions and shallots. They contain vitamins A and C, and the B vitamins, and they are a rich source of vitamin K.

PER SERVING: 407 CAL | 2.3G FAT | 0.7G SAT FAT | 73.4G CARBS | 27.2G SUGARS | 2.1G SALT | 10.2G FIBER | 25.5G PROTEIN

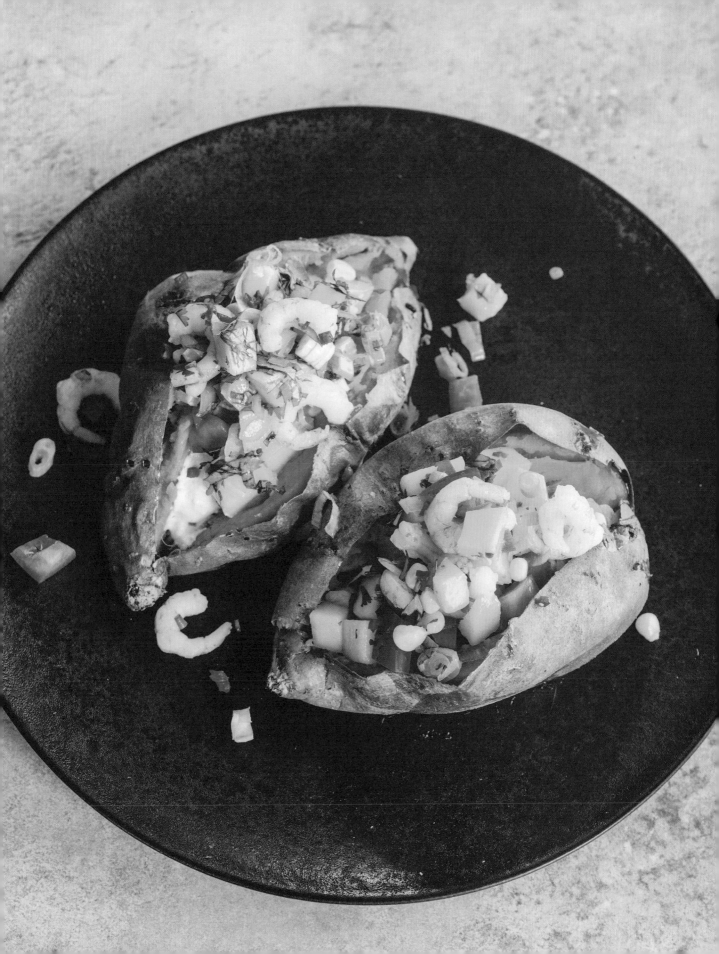

QUINOA SALAD WITH FENNEL AND ORANGE

Fennel is known to be an effective diuretic and calms the stomach, so it is a useful addition to any detox diet. It is delicious with zingy orange.

SERVES: 4 PREP: 20 MINS COOK: 15 MINS

3³/₄ cups vegetable stock
1¹/₃ cups quinoa, rinsed
3 oranges
1 fennel bulb, thinly sliced, green feathery tops reserved and torn into small pieces
2 scallions, finely chopped
¹/₄ cup coarsely chopped fresh flat-leaf parsley

DRESSING
juice of ¹/₂ lemon
3 tablespoons virgin olive oil
pepper, to taste

1 Bring the stock to a boil in a saucepan, add the quinoa, and simmer for 10–12 minutes, or until the germs separate from the seeds. Drain off the stock and discard, then spoon the quinoa into a salad bowl and let cool.

2 Grate the zest from two of the oranges and put it in a screw-top jar. Cut the peel and pith away from all three oranges with a small serrated knife. Hold each one above a bowl and cut between the membranes to release the segments into the bowl. Squeeze the juice from the membranes into the screw-top jar.

3 Add the orange segments, fennel slices, scallions, and parsley to the quinoa.

4 To make the dressing, add the lemon juice and oil to the screw-top jar, season with pepper, screw on the lid, and shake well. Drizzle the dressing over the salad and toss. Garnish with the feathery fennel tops and serve immediately.

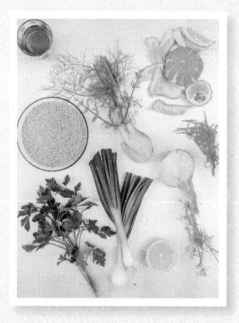

NUTRITIOUS QUINOA

Quinoa, pronounced "keen-wa," contains all eight essential amino acids, plus it's rich in fiber and minerals and lower in carbs than most grains.

PER SERVING: 388 CAL | 8.3G FAT | 1.9G SAT FAT | 54G CARBS | 11.6G SUGARS | 2.1G SALT | 8.4G FIBER | 10G PROTEIN

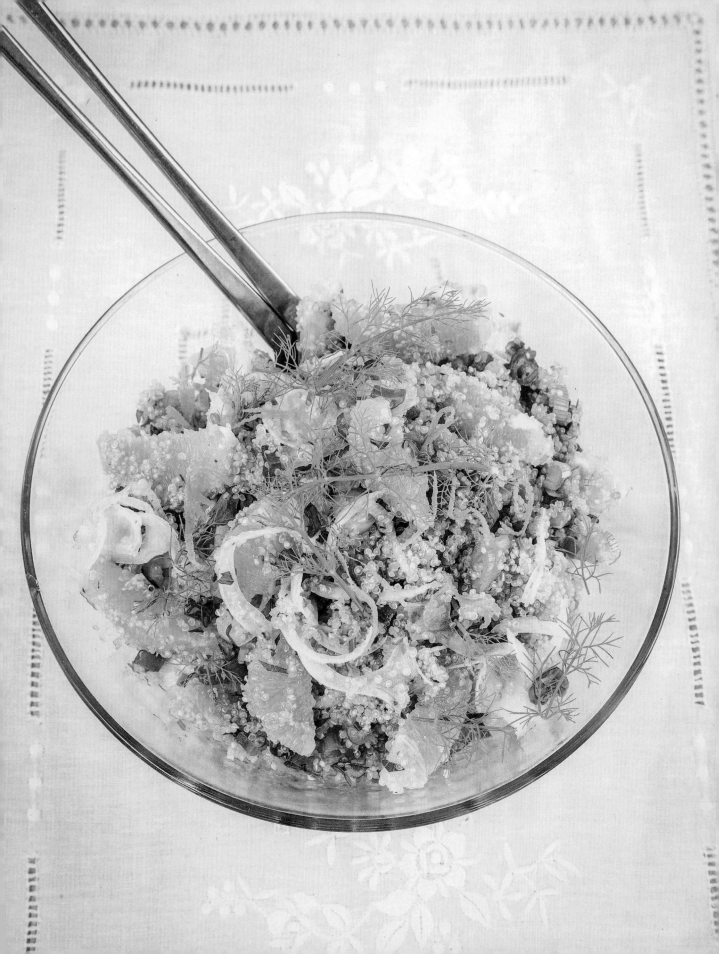

VIETNAMESE TOFU AND NOODLE SALAD

Packed with protein-boosting tofu and baby green edamame, this gingered salad is mixed with buckwheat noodles, making it a superfood feast.

SERVES: 4
PREP: 15 MINS, PLUS MARINATING   COOK: 8 MINS

14 ounces firm chilled tofu, drained and cut into 8 slices
4 ounces buckwheat soba noodles
1¹⁄₃ cups frozen edamame
1 carrot, cut into matchstick strips
1¹⁄₄ cups snow peas, cut into matchstick strips
4 ounces rainbow Swiss chard, stems cut into matchstick strips, leaves thinly shredded
¹⁄₃ cup coarsely chopped fresh cilantro

MARINADE
2 tablespoons tamari sauce or soy sauce
2 tablespoons sesame seeds
1 red chile, seeded and finely chopped (optional)
1¹⁄₂-inch piece fresh ginger, peeled and finely chopped

DRESSING
¹⁄₄ cup virgin canola oil
juice of ¹⁄₂ lemon
1 tablespoon sweet chili dipping sauce

1 Line the bottom of the broiler pan with aluminum foil. Arrange the tofu on the broiler pan in a single layer and fold up the edges of the foil to make a dish.

2 To make the marinade, mix together the tamari sauce, sesame seeds, chile, if using, and half the ginger in a small bowl. Spoon it over the tofu, then let marinate for 10 minutes.

3 Meanwhile, bring a large saucepan of water to a boil, add the noodles, and cook according to package directions, adding the frozen edamame for the last 3–4 minutes and cooking until just tender. Drain into a strainer, then rinse under cold running water.

4 Put the carrot, snow peas, Swiss chard stems and leaves, and cilantro in a large salad bowl. Add the noodles and edamame and gently toss.

5 To make the dressing, put the oil, lemon juice, sweet chili dipping sauce, and remaining ginger into a bowl and whisk with a fork. Pour over the salad and gently toss.

6 Preheat the broiler to medium–high. Turn the tofu over in the marinade, then broil for 2 minutes on each side, or until browned. Let cool for a few minutes, then cut into cubes and sprinkle over the salad with any remaining marinade and serve.

TERRIFIC TOFU

An everyday ingredient in Chinese and Thai cooking, tofu is made in much the same way that we make cheese, but using soy milk. It is rich in protein, vitamin E, calcium, iron, and other minerals, but low in fat. It is believed to alleviate the symptoms of menopause and help protect against heart disease.

PER SERVING: 483 CAL | 27.2G FAT | 2.6G SAT FAT | 34.5G CARBS | 6.1G SUGARS | 2.6G SALT | 8.3G FIBER | 28.8G PROTEIN

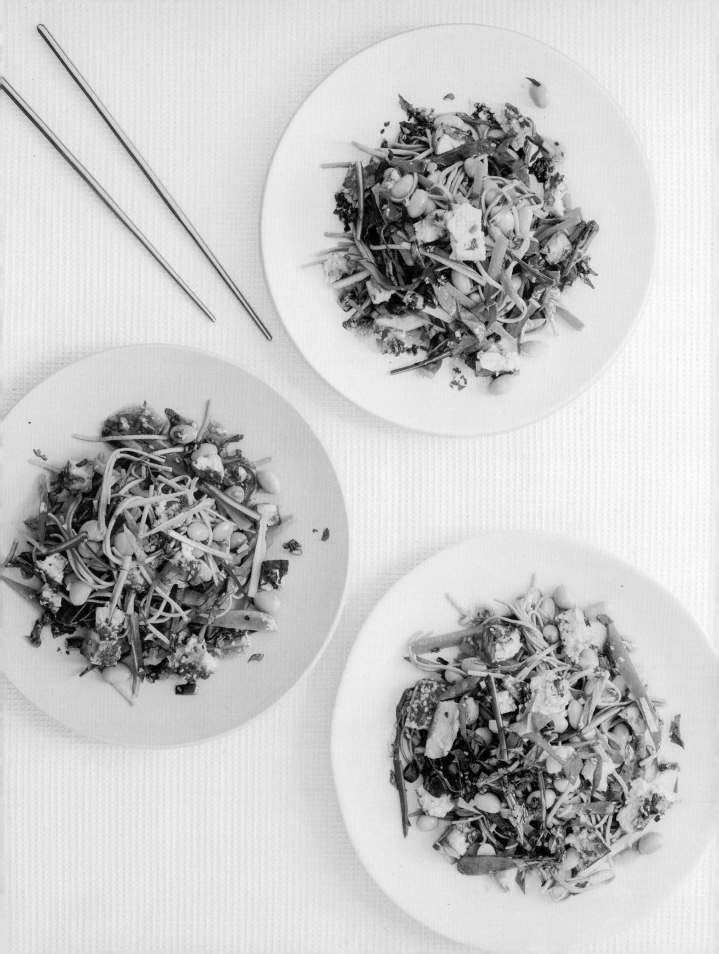

ROASTED BEET AND SQUASH SALAD

This nutty-tasting whole-grain salad, topped with two superfoods—beet and squash—can be made the night before, chilled, then tossed with beet leaves when serving.

SERVES: 4   PREP: 25 MINS   COOK: 30 MINS

5 raw beets (about 1 pound), cut into cubes
3 1/4 cups butternut squash cubes
1/4 cup virgin olive oil
1/2 cup long-grain brown rice
1/2 cup French red Camargue rice (available online), or another 1/2 cup long-grain brown rice
1/2 cup farro (emmer wheat) or pearl barley
4 cups baby beet leaves
salt and pepper, to taste

DRESSING
1 tablespoon flaxseed oil
2 tablespoons red wine vinegar
1/2 teaspoon smoked hot paprika
1 teaspoon fennel seeds, coarsely crushed
2 teaspoons tomato paste

1 Preheat the oven to 400°F. Put the beets and squash into a roasting pan, drizzle with half the olive oil, and season with salt and pepper. Roast for 30 minutes, or until just tender.

2 Meanwhile, bring a large saucepan of water to a boil, add the brown rice, red Camargue rice, and farro, and cook for about 30 minutes, or according to the package directions, until all the grains are tender. (Depending on the brand, one of the grains may need more cooking time then another; start with the grain that needs the longest cooking time, then add the other grains so they will have just enough cooking time to be tender but not overcooked.) Drain and rinse, then transfer to a plate.

3 To make the dressing, put all the ingredients and the remaining 2 tablespoons of olive oil in a screw-top jar, season with salt and pepper, screw on the lid, and shake well. Drizzle over the rice mixture, then toss gently together.

4 Spoon the roasted vegetables over the grains and let cool. Toss gently, then sprinkle with the beet leaves and serve immediately.

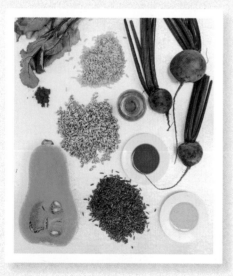

BEET BONANZA

Packed with vitamins, minerals, protein, energy-boosting carbs, and powerful antioxidants, beets are thought to help reduce the oxidation of LDL cholesterol, so reducing the risk of heart disease and stroke. They are also rich in potassium, folic acid, and iron.

PER SERVING: 505 CAL | 19.3G FAT | 2.5G SAT FAT | 75G CARBS | 10.7G SUGARS | 1.1G SALT | 9G FIBER | 10G PROTEIN

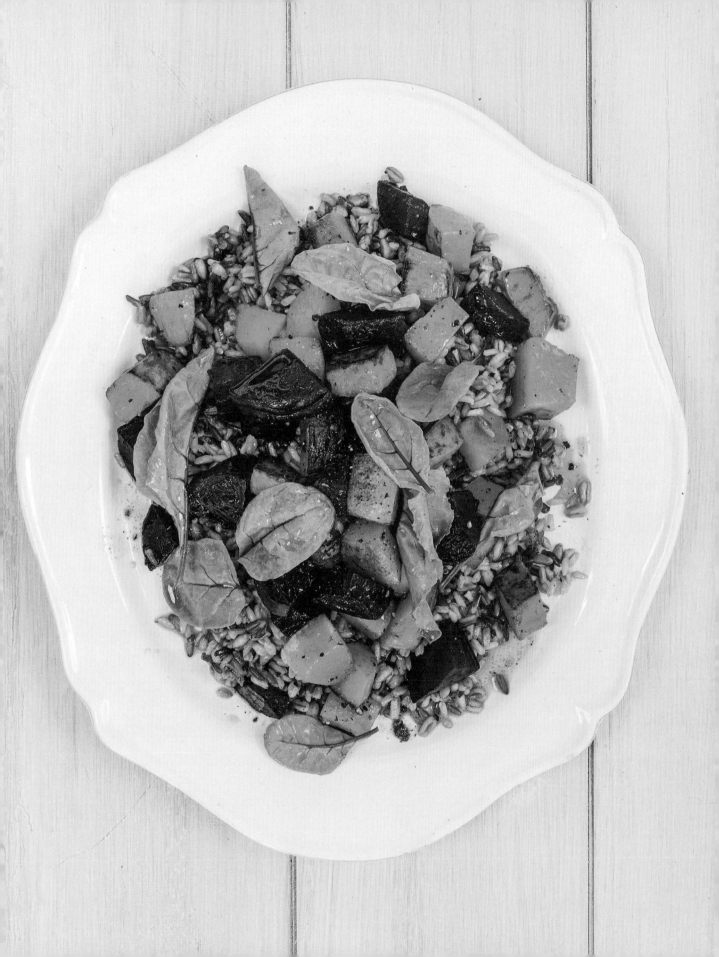

SUPERGREEN SALAD

Supercharged with vitamins and minerals, this crisp green salad tastes delicious with the addition of creamy smooth avocado and crunchy toasted seeds.

SERVES: 4   PREP: 15 MINS   COOK: 5 MINS

2 tablespoons pumpkin seeds
2 tablespoons sunflower seeds
2 tablespoons sesame seeds
4 teaspoons tamari sauce or soy sauce
3 1/2 cups broccoli florets
3 cups baby spinach
3/4 cup thinly shredded kale
1/3 cup coarsely chopped fresh cilantro
2 avocados, pitted, peeled, and sliced
juice of 2 limes

DRESSING
3 tablespoons flaxseed oil
2 teaspoons honey
pepper, to taste

1 Place a skillet over high heat. Add the pumpkin, sunflower, and sesame seeds, cover and dry-fry for 3–4 minutes, or until lightly toasted and beginning to pop, shaking the pan from time to time. Remove from the heat and stir in the tamari sauce.

2 Fill the bottom of a steamer halfway with water, bring to a boil, then put the broccoli in the steamer top, cover with a lid, and steam for 3–5 minutes, or until tender. Transfer to a salad bowl and add the spinach, kale, and cilantro.

3 Put the avocados and half the lime juice in a small bowl and toss well, then transfer to the salad bowl.

4 To make the dressing, put the remaining lime juice, the oil, honey, and a little pepper in a small bowl and whisk together with a fork. Sprinkle the toasted seeds over the salad and serve immediately with the dressing for pouring over the top.

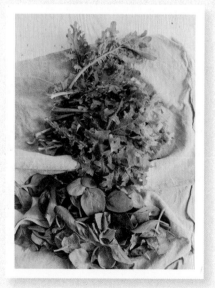

GO GREEN

Spinach, kale, and broccoli contain beneficial phytochemicals that help to prevent carcinogens from damaging DNA and so help to protect against cancer. They are also rich in vitamins A and C, the B vitamins, and iron.

PER SERVING: 388 CAL | 32.8G FAT | 3.9G SAT FAT | 22.1G CARBS | 5G SUGARS | 0.9G SALT | 10.7G FIBER | 9G PROTEIN

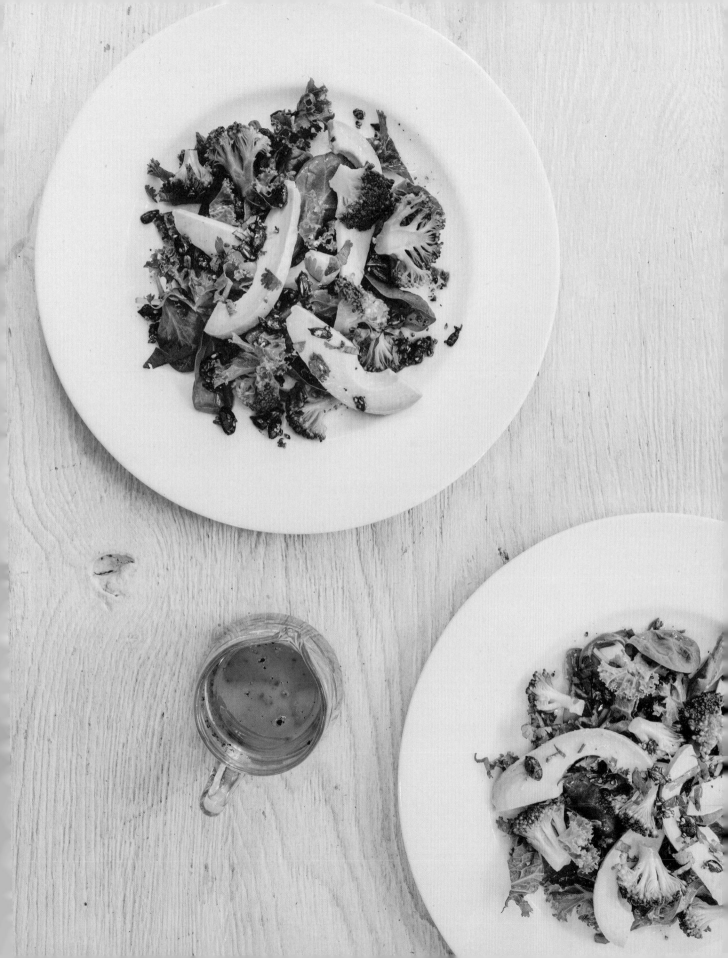

CRANBERRY AND RED CABBAGE COLESLAW

Forget about coleslaw coated in thick, high-calorie mayonnaise. This version is tossed with a tangy orange and olive oil dressing flavored with chia seeds and toasted walnuts.

SERVES: 4   PREP: 15 MINS   COOK: 3 MINS

1½ cups thinly shredded red cabbage
1 carrot, shredded
1 cup cauliflower florets
1 red-skinned sweet, crisp apple, quartered, cored, and thinly sliced
⅓ cup dried cranberries
1 cup alfalfa and sango radish sprouts

DRESSING
⅓ cup coarsely chopped walnuts
juice of 1 orange
¼ cup virgin olive oil
2 tablespoons chia seeds
salt and pepper, to taste

1 Put the red cabbage, carrot, and cauliflower into a salad bowl. Add the apple, dried cranberries, and sprouts and toss well.

2 To make the dressing, put the walnuts in a large skillet and toast for 2–3 minutes, or until just beginning to brown.

3 Put the orange juice, oil, and chia seeds in a small bowl, season with salt and pepper, then stir in the hot walnuts. Pour the dressing over the salad and toss. Serve immediately or cover and chill in the refrigerator until needed.

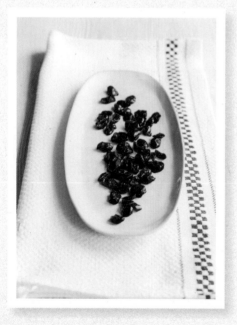

HEALTHY CRANBERRIES

Cranberries are packed with antioxidants. They are believed to help reduce inflammation and to be a useful tool in the fight against heart disease.

PER SERVING: 320 CAL | 23.2G FAT | 2.8G SAT FAT | 29.5G CARBS | 16G SUGARS | 0.8G SALT | 9.3G FIBER | 4.9G PROTEIN

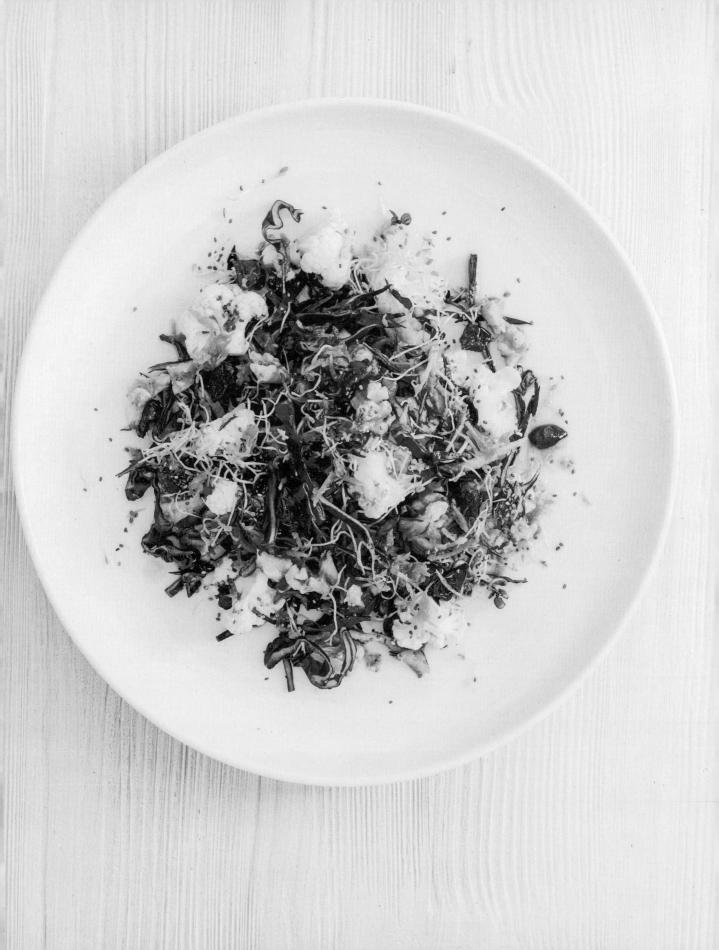

SWEET POTATO FRIES

A sunshine snack, Caribbean-style. Replace the oil spray with vegetable oil if you prefer, but heat it in the oven before adding the sweet potatoes.

SERVES: 4   PREP: 15 MINS   COOK: 20 MINS

2 squirts of vegetable oil spray
6 sweet potatoes (about 2 pounds)
1/2 teaspoon salt
1/2 teaspoon ground cumin
1/4 teaspoon cayenne pepper

1 Preheat the oven to 450°F. Spray a large baking pan with vegetable oil spray.

2 Cut the sweet potatoes into 1/4-inch-thick sticks. Arrange them in the prepared baking pan in a single layer and spray with vegetable oil spray.

3 Mix together the salt, cumin, and cayenne pepper in a small bowl, then sprinkle the mixture evenly over the sweet potatoes and toss well.

4 Bake for 15–20 minutes, or until cooked through and lightly browned. Serve hot.

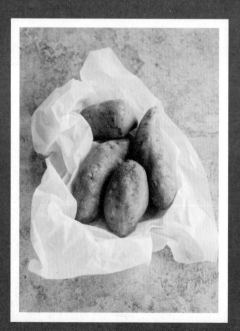

SWEET POTATOES

Loaded with vitamins A and C, fiber, and potassium, sweet potatoes are a terrific superfood. They also contain cancer-fighting antioxidants and useful amounts of magnesium and manganese.

PER SERVING: 194 CAL | 0.1G FAT | TRACE SAT FAT | 45.2 CARBS | 9.4G SUGARS | 1G SALT | 6.7G FIBER | 3.5G PROTEIN

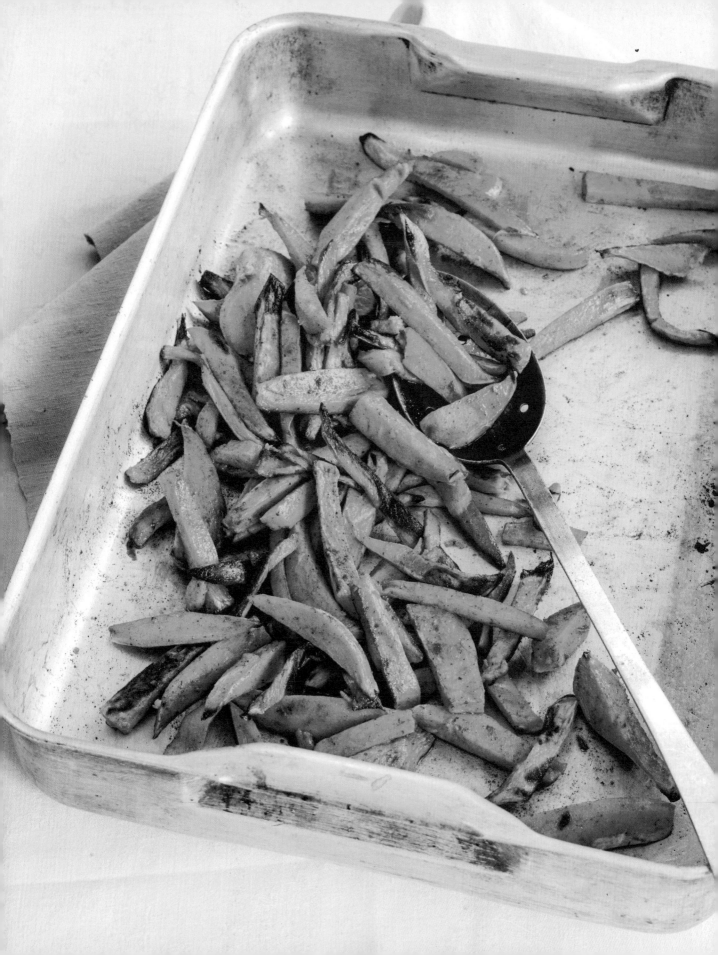

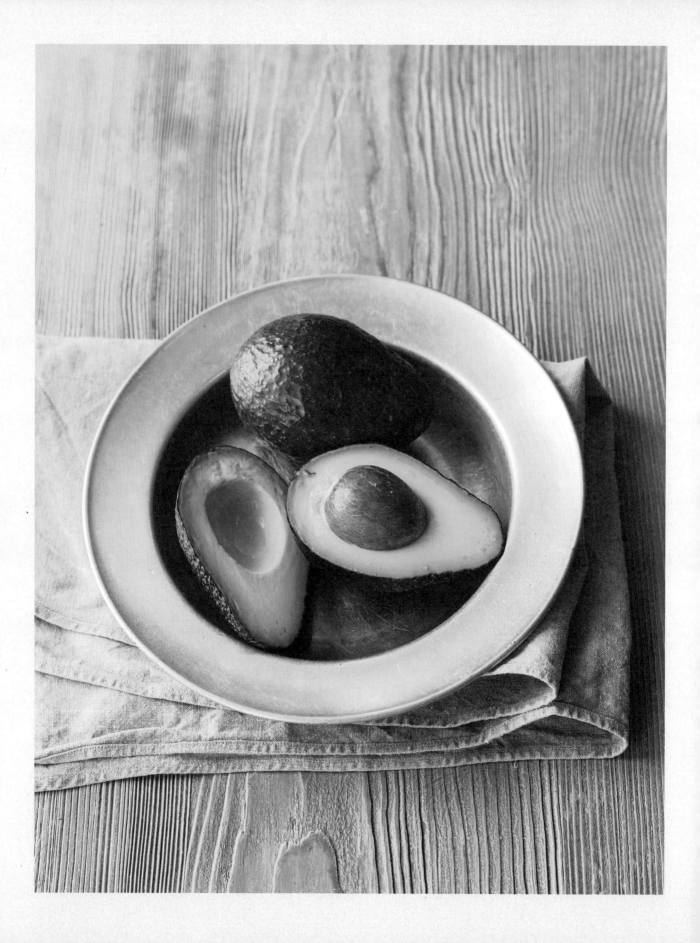

GUACAMOLE DIP

A Mexican-style dip that is delicious with raw, nutrition-packed vegetable sticks and hot pita breads.

SERVES: 4   PREP: 10 MINS

2 large avocados, pitted, peeled, and sliced
juice of 2 limes
2 large garlic cloves, crushed
1 teaspoon mild chili powder, plus extra to garnish
salt and pepper

1 Put the avocado slices, lime juice, garlic, and chili powder in a food processor and process until smooth. Season with salt and pepper.

2 Transfer to a serving bowl, garnish with chili powder, and serve immediately.

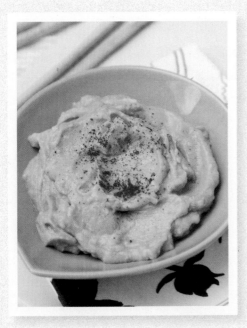

AMAZING AVOCADOS

Avocados are high in vitamin C and potassium, and contain healthy monounsaturated fats. They are an excellent source of vitamin E, which helps keep the heart healthy, and contain good amounts of vitamin B_6, which is essential for a healthy nervous system.

PER SERVING: 170 CAL | 14.7G FAT | 2.1G SAT FAT | 11.1G CARBS | 1.1G SUGARS | 0.8G SALT | 7.1G FIBER | 2.3G PROTEIN

POWER BALLS

Packed with superfoods, these truffle-size balls are a mighty mixture of slow-release carbohydrates, protein, and minerals. They're great for lunch bags in place of chocolate.

MAKES: 20 BALLS   PREP: 25 MINS

3 ounces semisweet chocolate
1/4 cup sunflower seeds
1/4 cup flaxseed
1/4 cup sesame seeds
3/4 cup Brazil nuts, coarsely chopped
6 Medjool dates, pitted
1/3 cup dried goji berries
1 teaspoon ground cinnamon
1 tablespoon maca (see page 16)
1/2 cup dry unsweetened coconut flakes
1/3 cup plus 1 tablespoon maple syrup

1 Break 2 ounces of the chocolate into pieces and reserve the rest. Put the sunflower seeds, flaxseed, sesame seeds, Brazil nuts, and chocolate into a food processor and process until finely ground, scraping down the sides of the processor once or twice.

2 Add the dates, goji berries, cinnamon, maca, and 1/3 cup of the coconut, then spoon in the maple syrup. Process until you have a coarse paste.

3 Using a measuring spoon, scoop out tablespoons of the mixture onto a plate, then shape them to make 20 mounds. Roll them into balls.

4 Put the remaining coconut on one plate and finely grate the remaining chocolate onto another plate. Roll half the balls in the coconut and the rest in the chocolate. Pack into an airtight container and store in the refrigerator for up to three days.

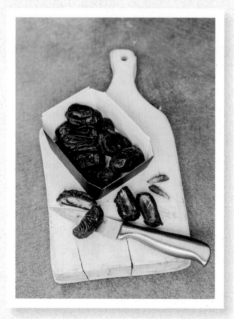

DATES FOR FIBER

Dates are high in fiber and are a good source of potassium, calcium, iron, phosphorus, manganese, copper, and magnesium. They are thought to help prevent some cancers and intestinal diseases.

PER BALL: 132 CAL | 7.7G FAT | 2.4G SAT FAT | 15.2G CARBS | 10.9G SUGARS | TRACE SALT | 2.4G FIBER | 2.1G PROTEIN

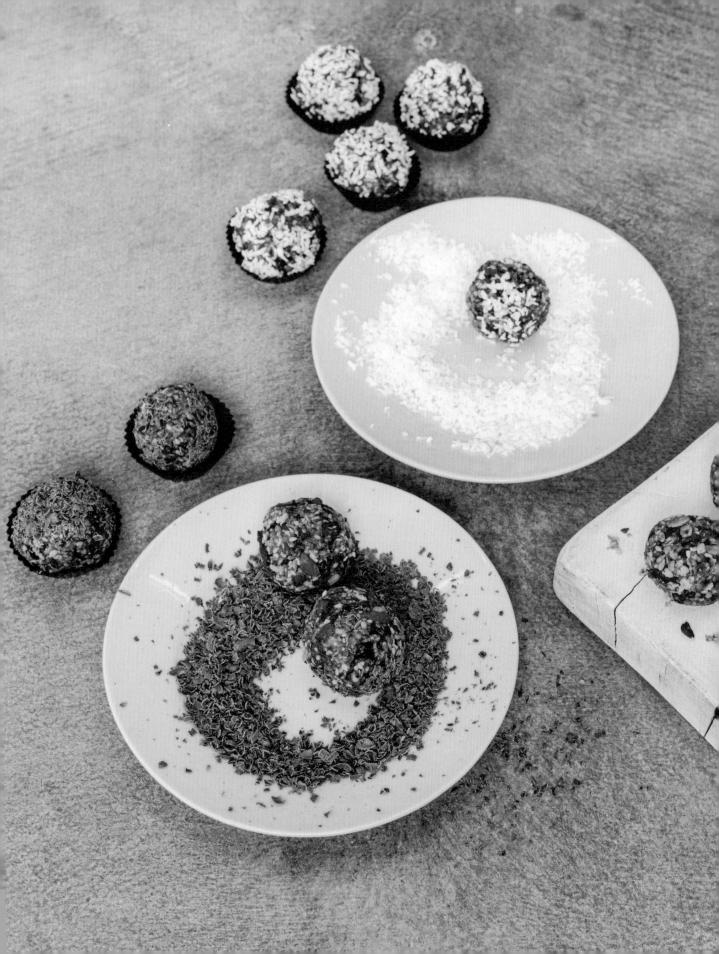

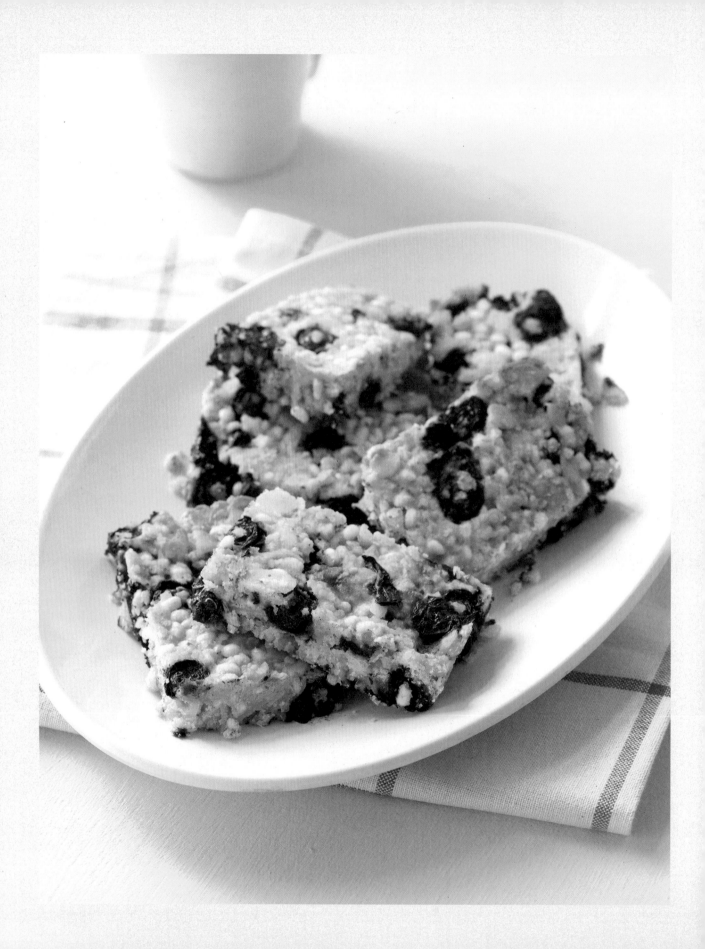

HONEY AND BLUEBERRY BARS

*Honey gives cakes and baked goods a rich flavor and chewy texture.
These portable snacks are ideal for packing ahead of a long journey.*

MAKES: 12 BARS
PREP: 15 MINS   COOK: 30 MINS, PLUS COOLING

sunflower oil, to grease
2/3 cup all-purpose flour sifted with
1/2 teaspoon baking powder
1/2 cup quinoa flakes
3 2/3 cups puffed rice
1/2 cup slivered almonds
1 1/2 cups blueberries
1 stick butter
1/3 cup plus 1 tablespoon honey
1 egg, beaten

1 Preheat the oven to 350°F. Brush a shallow 11 x 7-inch baking pan with oil and line the bottom with parchment paper.

2 Mix together the flour and baking powder mixture, quinoa flakes, puffed rice, almonds, and blueberries in a bowl.

3 Heat the butter and honey in a saucepan over low heat until melted, then pour over the dry ingredients. Add the egg, and stir well.

4 Spoon the batter into the prepared pan and level with a spatula. Bake for 25–30 minutes, or until golden brown and firm. Let cool in the pan for 15 minutes, then cut into 12 bars and transfer to a wire rack to cool completely.

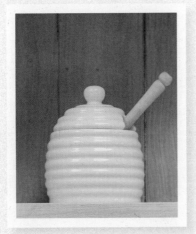

HEAVENLY HONEY

Honey is a natural sweetener that has long been praised for its antibacterial properties.

PER BAR: 182 CAL | 9.3G FAT | 1.6G SAT FAT | 22.9G CARBS | 9.2G SUGARS | 0.1G SALT | 1.5G FIBER | 3G PROTEIN

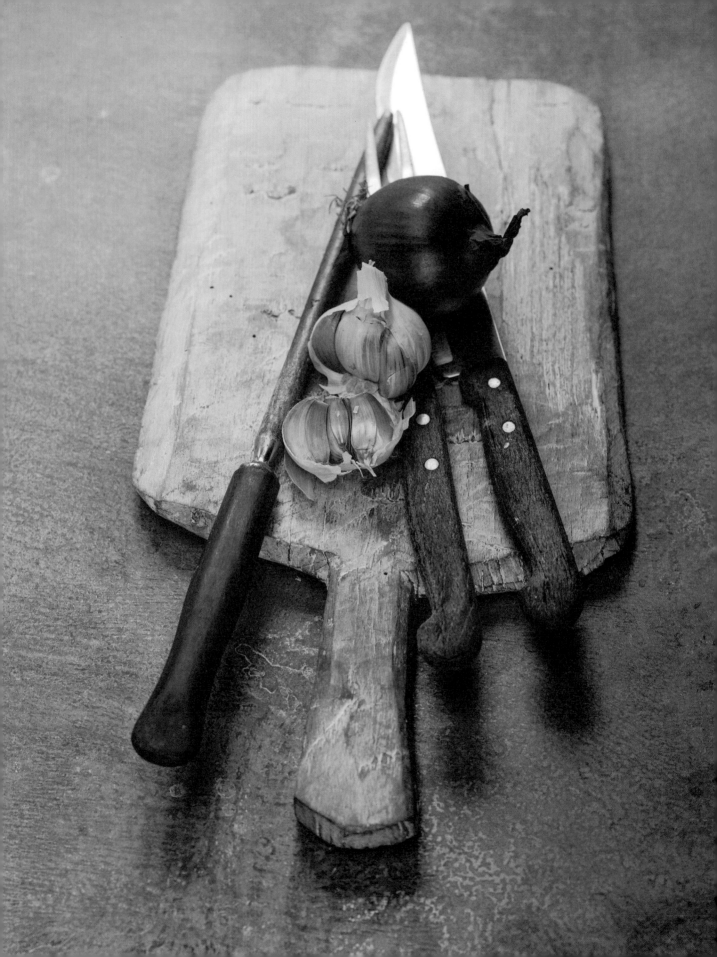

MAIN DISHES

Beef stir-fry   74

Pork medallions with pomegranate salad   76

Jerk chicken with papaya and avocado salsa   78

Spicy roasted turkey   80

Tangy turkey meatballs with edamame   82

Broiled trout stuffed with spinach and mushrooms   85

Gingered salmon with stir-fried kale   86

Broiled salmon with mango and lime salsa   88

Risotto primavera   90

Beet burgers in buns   93

Stuffed red peppers   94

Black bean and quinoa burritos   97

Raw sprouts and seeds supersalad   98

BEEF STIR-FRY

Beef is high in iron and the vegetables in this dish are rich in vitamin C, which helps us to absorb the iron, making it a great combination.

SERVES: 2   PREP: 10 MINS   COOK: 12 MINS

2 teaspoons olive oil
5 ounces top sirloin steak, visible fat removed, cut into thin strips
1 orange bell pepper, seeded and cut into thin strips
4 scallions, finely chopped
1–2 fresh jalapeño chiles, seeded and thinly sliced
2 garlic cloves, finely chopped
2 cups snow peas, halved diagonally
4 ounces large portobello mushrooms, sliced
2 teaspoons hoisin sauce
1 tablespoon orange juice
5 cups arugula or watercress
4 tablespoons sweet chili dipping sauce, to serve

1 Heat the oil in a wok over medium–high heat for 30 seconds. Add the beef and stir-fry for 1 minute, or until browned. Transfer to a plate with a slotted spoon.

2 Add the orange bell pepper, scallions, jalapeño chiles, and garlic to the wok and stir-fry for 2 minutes. Add the snow peas and mushrooms and stir-fry for an additional 2 minutes.

3 Return the beef to the wok. Add the hoisin sauce and orange juice and stir-fry for 2–3 minutes, or until the beef is cooked and the vegetables are tender but still firm. Add the arugula and stir-fry until it starts to wilt. Serve immediately with a small bowl of sweet chili dipping sauce.

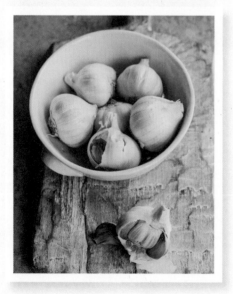

GREAT GARLIC

Garlic is considered to have anti-inflammatory properties, as well as antibacterial and antiviral benefits. It is believed to help lower cholesterol and blood pressure.

PER SERVING: 160 CAL | 3G FAT | 1G SAT FAT | 9G CARBS | 8G SUGARS | 0.8G SALT | 5G FIBER | 20G PROTEIN

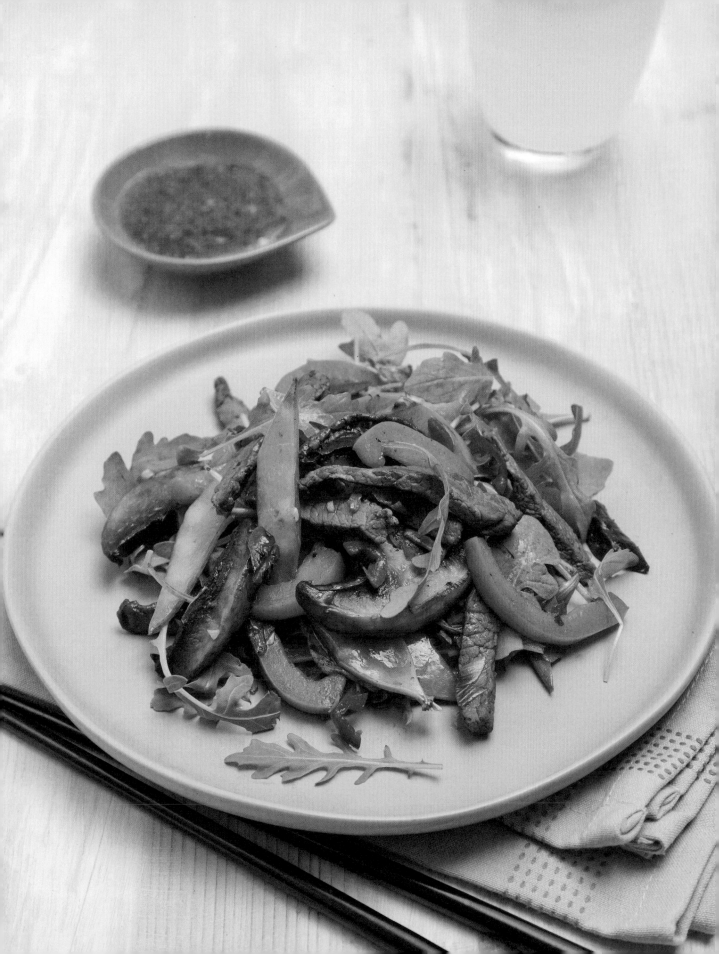

PORK MEDALLIONS WITH POMEGRANATE SALAD

Fresh herbs and jewel-like pomegranate give this nutritious salad a delicious Middle Eastern flavor.

SERVES: 4 PREP: 10 MINS COOK: 30 MINS

³/4 cup wheat berries
¹/3 cup coarsely chopped fresh flat-leaf parsley
³/4 cup thinly shredded kale
seeds of 1 pomegranate
1 tablespoon olive oil
4 (4¹/2-ounce) pork medallions, visible fat removed
2 garlic cloves, finely chopped
salt and pepper, to taste

DRESSING
¹/3 cup coarsely chopped walnuts
3 tablespoons virgin olive oil
1 tablespoon pomegranate molasses
juice of 1 lemon

1 Bring a medium saucepan of water to a boil. Add the wheat berries and simmer for 25–30 minutes, or according to package directions, until tender. Drain and rinse.

2 Meanwhile, to make the dressing, put the walnuts in a large skillet and toast for 2–3 minutes, or until just beginning to brown. Put the virgin olive oil, pomegranate molasses, and lemon juice into a small bowl and mix together with a fork. Season with salt and pepper and stir in the hot walnuts.

3 Mix together the parsley, kale, and pomegranate seeds in a large bowl.

4 Heat the olive oil in the skillet over medium heat. Add the pork and garlic, season with salt and pepper, and cook for 10 minutes, turning halfway through, until browned and cooked. Cut into the center of one of the pork medallions; any juices that run out should be clear and piping hot with steam rising. Slice the pork into strips.

5 Add the wheat berries to the kale and gently toss. Transfer to a plate, pour the dressing over the grains and vegetables, then top with the pork and serve.

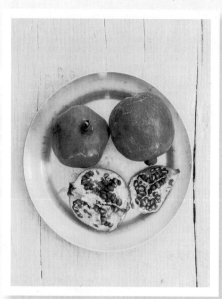

PREPARING POMEGRANATES

Cut through the hard outer casing of a pomegranate to reveal the closely packed ruby seeds that are rich in vitamins A, C, and E plus antioxidants. Break and flex the fruit to pop out the seeds, or turn upside-down over a bowl and hit the rounded edge with a wooden spoon to knock them out.

PER SERVING: 540 CAL | 29.7G FAT | 5.2G SAT FAT | 37G CARBS | 4.5G SUGARS | 0.9G SALT | 6.9G FIBER | 34.6G PROTEIN

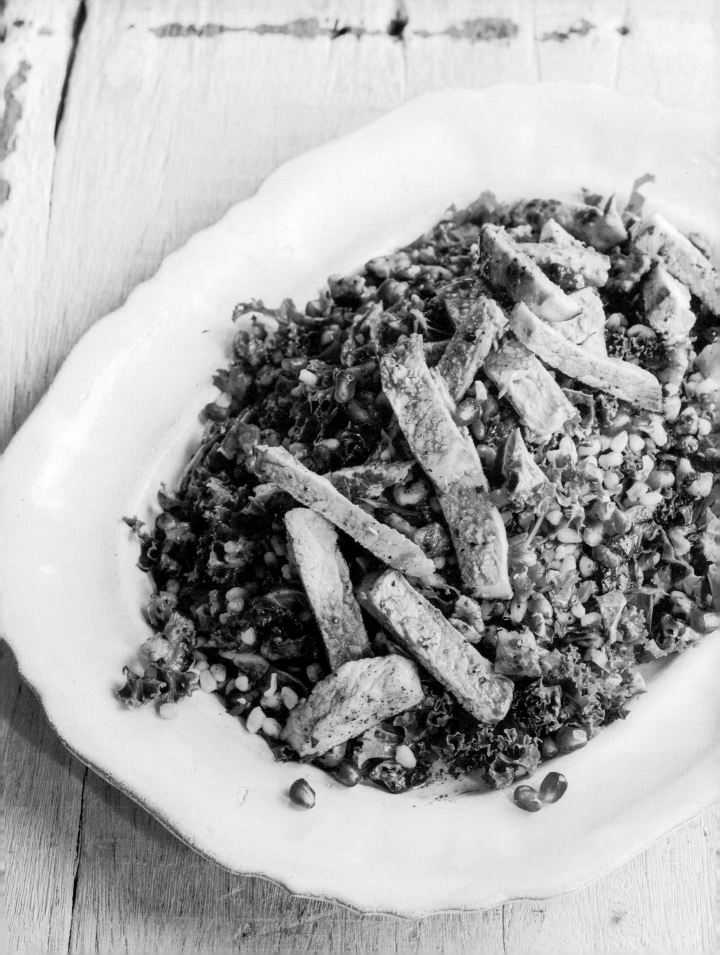

JERK CHICKEN WITH PAPAYA AND AVOCADO SALSA

*Glazed chicken doesn't need to have a high-calorie coating,
as this flavor-packed Jamaican dry spice rub shows.*

SERVES: 4   PREP: 15 MINS   COOK: 35 MINS

2¼ pounds small chicken drumsticks, skinned
1 tablespoon olive oil
1 romaine lettuce, leaves separated and torn into pieces (optional)
3 cups baby spinach (optional)

JERK SPICE RUB
1 teaspoon allspice berries, crushed
1 teaspoon coriander seeds, crushed
1 teaspoon mild paprika
¼ teaspoon freshly grated nutmeg
1 tablespoon fresh thyme leaves
1 tablespoon black peppercorns, coarsely crushed
pinch of salt

PAPAYA AND AVOCADO SALSA
1 papaya, halved, seeded, peeled, and cut into cubes
2 large avocados, pitted, peeled, and cut into cubes
finely grated zest and juice of 1 lime
½ red chile, seeded and finely chopped
½ red onion, finely chopped
⅓ cup fresh cilantro, finely chopped
2 teaspoons chia seeds

1   Preheat the oven to 400°F. To make the jerk spice rub, mix together all the ingredients in a small bowl.

2   Slash each chicken drumstick two or three times with a knife, then put them in a roasting pan and drizzle with the oil. Sprinkle the spice mix over the chicken, then rub it in with your fingers, washing your hands well afterwards. Roast the chicken for 30–35 minutes, or until browned with piping hot juices that run clear with no sign of pink when the tip of a sharp knife is inserted into the thickest part of a drumstick.

3   Meanwhile, to make the salsa, put the papaya and avocados in a bowl, sprinkle with the lime zest and juice, then toss well. Add the chile, red onion, cilantro, and chia seeds and stir.

4   Toss the lettuce and spinach together, if using. Serve with the chicken and salsa.

THREE CHEERS FOR CHIA

Chia is a good source of omega-3 fats and fiber, and it contains calcium, manganese, and phosphorus. It is thought to have many health benefits, including providing energy, stabilizing blood sugar, aiding digestion, and lowering cholesterol.

PER SERVING: 394 CAL | 18.1G FAT | 3.2G SAT FAT | 17.1G CARBS | 5.4G SUGARS | 0.9G SALT | 7.8G FIBER | 42G PROTEIN

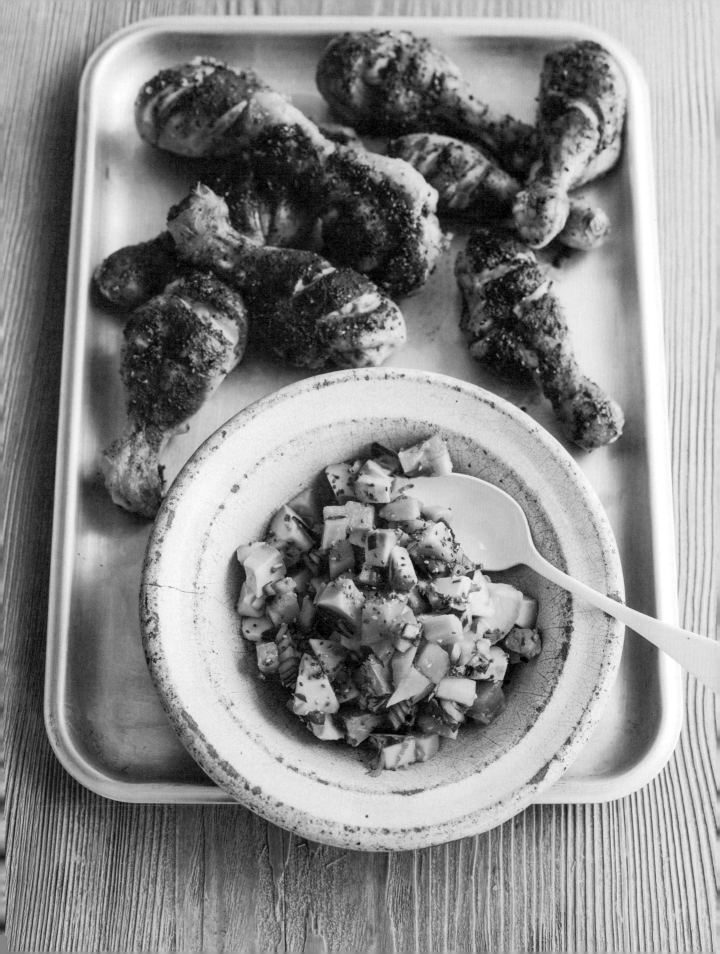

SPICY ROASTED TURKEY

*This easy one-dish meal makes a healthy midweek dinner—
with little dishwashing required.*

SERVES: 4   PREP: 20 MINS   COOK: 45 MINS

3 tablespoons olive oil
1/2 butternut squash or other squash (about 1 pound),
seeded, peeled, and cut into large pieces
3 sweet potatoes, cut into large pieces
7 ounces baby carrots, tops trimmed, larger ones
halved lengthwise
1 small cauliflower, cut into large florets
1 pound skinless and boneless turkey breast,
cut into 1/2-inch-thick slices
salt and pepper, to taste

SPICE BLEND
2 tablespoons sesame seeds
2 tablespoons sunflower seeds
2 teaspoons mild paprika
1 teaspoon coriander seeds, crushed
1 teaspoon fennel seeds, crushed
1 teaspoon cumin seeds, crushed

1   Preheat the oven to 400°F. To make the spice blend, mix all the ingredients together in a small bowl and season with salt and pepper.

2   Pour the oil into a large roasting pan, then heat in the oven for 1 minute. Put the squash, sweet potatoes, and carrots in the roasting pan and toss in the hot oil. Roast for 15 minutes.

3   Add the cauliflower to the roasting pan and turn all the vegetables so they are coated in the oil. Push them to the edges of the pan, then add the turkey in a single layer.

4   Sprinkle the spice blend over the turkey and vegetables, then turn the vegetables so they are evenly coated. Roast for 20–25 minutes, or until the vegetables are tender and the turkey is golden brown with piping hot juices that run clear with no sign of pink when the thickest slice is cut in half.

5   Spoon the turkey and vegetables onto plates and serve immediately.

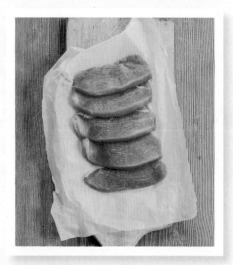

TALKING TURKEY

Turkey is a rich source of protein, but is low in fat. It also contains iron, zinc, potassium, and phosphorus, as well as vitamin B_6 and niacin, which are essential for the body's energy production.

PER SERVING: 455 CAL | 16.6G FAT | 2.3G SAT FAT | 45.5G CARBS | 11G SUGARS | 1.1G SALT | 9.8G FIBER | 34.2G PROTEIN

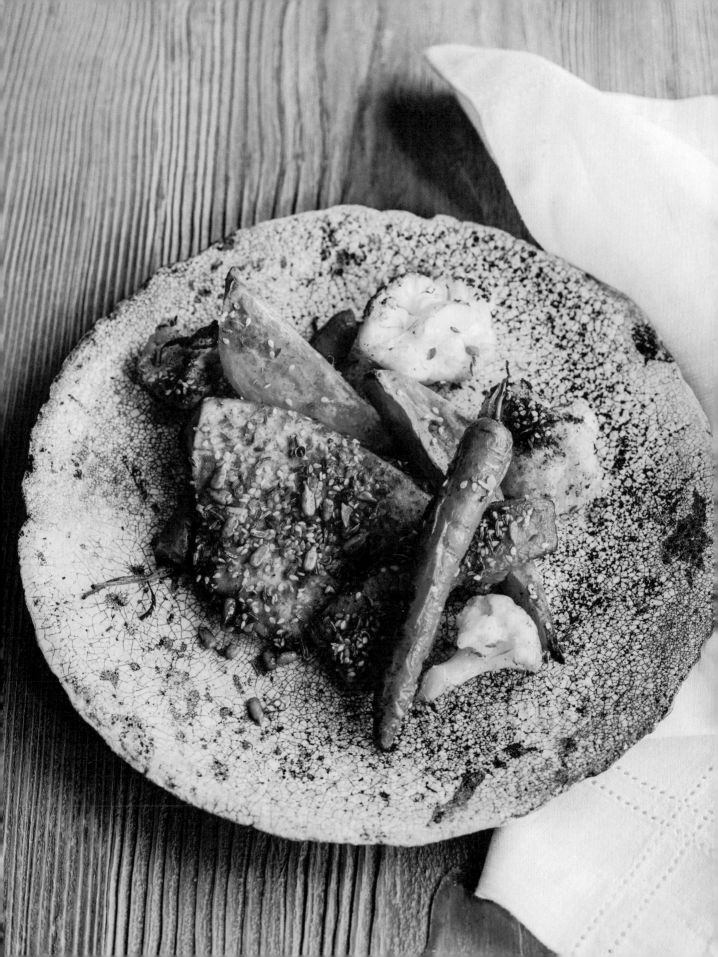

TANGY TURKEY MEATBALLS WITH EDAMAME

Ground turkey breast can be quickly processed with lemon and garlic to make this simple midweek dinner that's superhealthy, low in fat, and high in protein.

SERVES: 4   PREP: 20 MINS   COOK: 30 MINS

1¼ cups short-grain brown rice
1 small onion, coarsely chopped
1 slice of whole wheat bread, torn into pieces
2 garlic cloves, thinly sliced
1 pound ground turkey breast
finely grated zest of 1 unwaxed lemon
1 tablespoon olive oil
1½ cups chicken stock
1 cup frozen edamame
¾ cup peas
2 egg yolks
¼ cup coarsely chopped fresh flat-leaf parsley
⅓ cup coarsely chopped fresh mint
salt and pepper, to taste

1   Cook the rice in a large saucepan of lightly salted boiling water for 30 minutes, or according to the package directions, until tender. Drain well.

2   Meanwhile, put the onion, bread, and garlic in a food processor and process until finely chopped. Add the turkey and lemon zest and season with salt and pepper, then process again briefly until mixed.

3   Spoon the mixture into 20 mounds, then shape them into balls using wet hands.

4   Heat the oil in a large lidded skillet over medium heat. Add the meatballs in a single layer and cook for 15 minutes, or until evenly browned, turning from time to time.

5   Add the stock, cover, and cook for 5 minutes. Add the edamame and peas, replace the lid, and cook for 5 minutes, or until the vegetables are just tender and the meatballs are cooked through with juices that are piping hot and that run clear with no sign of pink when a meatball is cut in half. Remove from the heat and spoon the stock into a bowl.

6   Meanwhile, whisk the egg yolks together in a large bowl and season with salt and pepper. Gradually whisk in the stock until smooth, then pour the mixture back into the pan. Place over low heat and cook, stirring all the time, for 3–4 minutes, or until thickened. Be careful not to have the heat too high or the egg yolks will scramble.

7   Stir in the herbs. Spoon the rice into shallow bowls, top with the meatballs and sauce, and serve immediately.

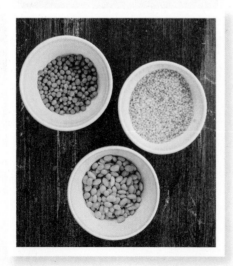

BEAUTIFUL BROWN RICE

Brown rice is unrefined, so it still has the hull and bran, making it rich in fiber, the B vitamins, magnesium, and potassium.

PER SERVING: 546 CAL | 11.8G FAT | 2.4G SAT FAT | 62.4G CARBS | 3.4G SUGARS | 1.8G SALT | 6.5G FIBER | 45G PROTEIN

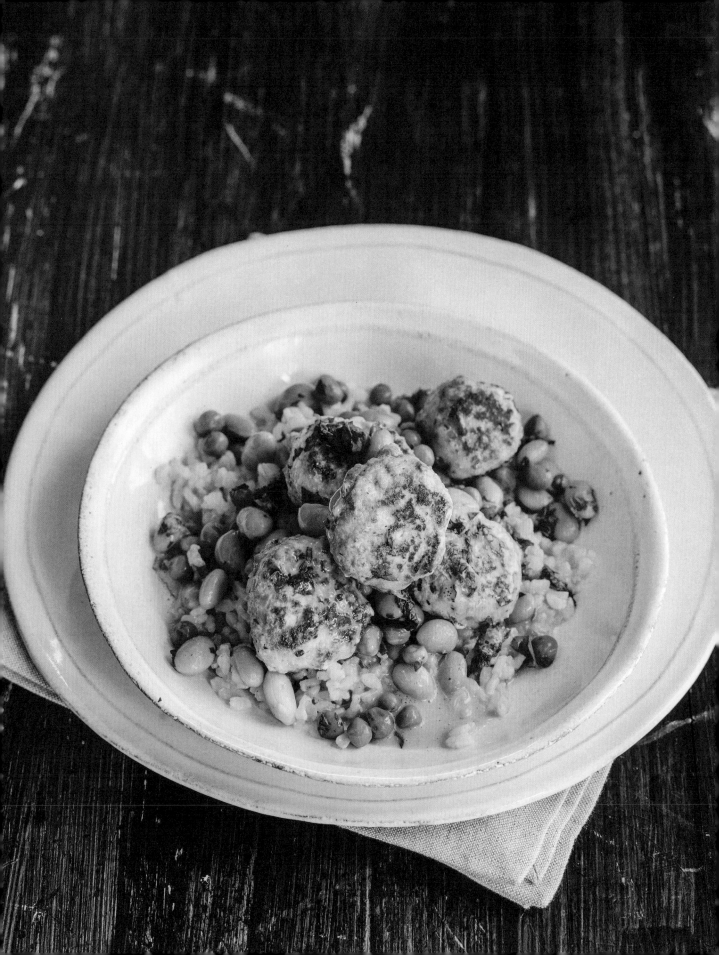

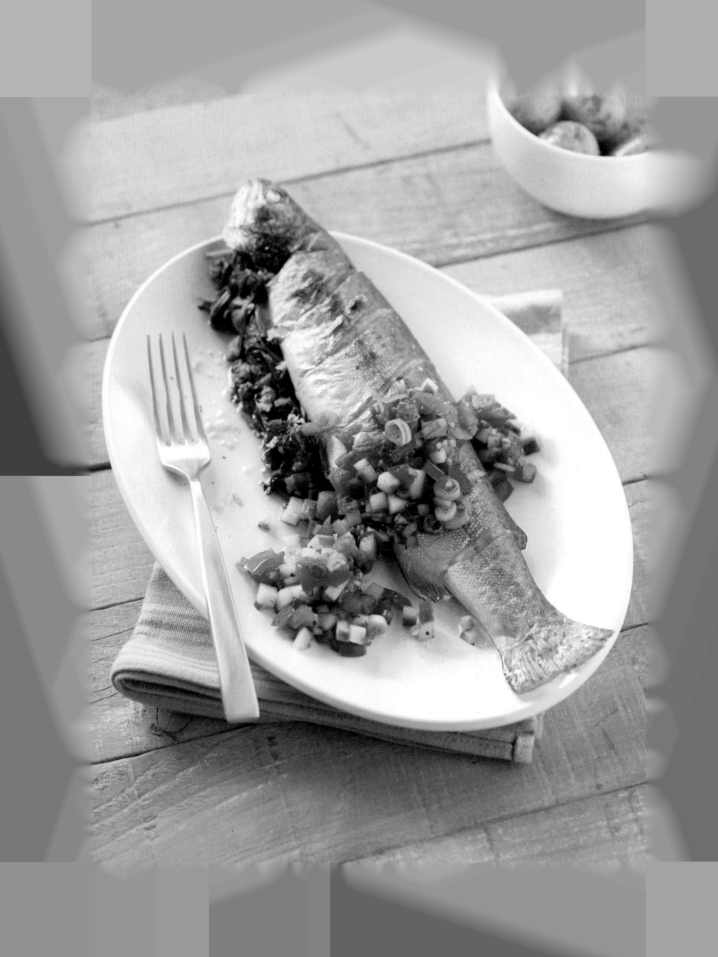

BROILED TROUT STUFFED WITH SPINACH AND MUSHROOMS

This glamorous-looking dish is a great way to power up on omega-3-rich oily fish while enjoying a delicious dinner for two.

SERVES: 2 PREP: 30 MINS COOK: 20 MINS

2 (12-ounce) trout, gutted and fins removed
1 tablespoon vegetable oil
1 pound new potatoes, boiled, to serve (optional)
salt and pepper, to taste

STUFFING
2 tablespoons butter
2 shallots, finely chopped
3/4 cup finely chopped mushrooms
2 cups baby spinach
1 tablespoon chopped fresh flat-leaf parsley
or tarragon
finely grated zest of 1 unwaxed lemon
grating of fresh nutmeg

TOMATO SALSA
2 tomatoes, peeled, seeded, and finely chopped
4-inch piece of cucumber, finely chopped
2 scallions, finely chopped
1 tablespoon olive oil

1 Rinse the trout inside and out under cold running water, then pat dry with paper towels. Slash the skin of each fish on both sides about five times with a knife. Brush with the oil and season well inside and out with salt and pepper.

2 To make the stuffing, melt the butter in a small saucepan over medium-low heat. Add the shallots and sauté for 2–3 minutes. Add the mushrooms and sauté for 2 minutes. Add the spinach and cook for 2–3 minutes, or until it has just wilted. Remove from the heat and stir in the parsley, lemon zest, and a good grating of nutmeg. Let cool.

3 Preheat the broiler to medium–high. Line the broiler rack with aluminum foil. Fill the cavities of the trout with the stuffing, then reshape them.

4 Broil the trout, turning halfway through, for 10–12 minutes, or until it flakes easily when pressed with a knife.

5 Meanwhile, to make the tomato salsa, mix together all the ingredients and season well with salt and pepper.

6 Serve the trout with the salsa spooned over, with the new potatoes, if using.

TASTY TROUT

Trout is rich in omega-3 fatty acids, which studies show help to reduce the risk of heart disease and strokes.

PER SERVING: 551 CAL | 36.5G FAT | 11.2G SAT FAT | 13G CARBS | 4.4G SUGARS | 3.5G SALT | 3.1G FIBER | 43.4G PROTEIN

GINGERED SALMON WITH STIR-FRIED KALE

A stir-fry is a great way of making sure you pack fresh vegetables into your diet, and this one is low in calories and carbohydrates.

SERVES: 4 PREP: 20 MINS COOK: 10 MINS

4 (5¹/2-ounce) salmon steaks, skinned
2-inch piece fresh ginger, peeled and
finely chopped
3 garlic cloves, finely chopped
1 red chile, seeded and finely chopped
3 tablespoons tamari sauce or soy sauce
3 cups broccoli florets
¹/3 cup water
1 tablespoon sunflower oil
1 large leek, sliced
2 cups thinly shredded kale
2 tablespoons Chinese rice wine
juice of 1 orange

1 Preheat the broiler to medium–high and line the bottom of the broiler pan with aluminum foil. Arrange the salmon on the broiler pan and fold up the edges of the foil to make a dish. Sprinkle over half the ginger, half the garlic, and half the chile, then drizzle with 1 tablespoon of tamari sauce. Broil, turning once, for 8–10 minutes, or until browned and the fish flakes easily when pressed with a knife.

2 Meanwhile, put the broccoli and water into a wok or large skillet, cover, and cook over medium–high heat for 3–4 minutes, or until the broccoli is almost tender. Pour off any remaining water.

3 Add the oil to the wok and increase the heat to high. When it is hot, add the leek and kale with the remaining ginger, garlic, and chile and stir-fry for 2–3 minutes, or until the kale has just wilted.

4 Mix in the remaining tamari sauce, the Chinese rice wine, and orange juice and cook for an additional 1 minute. Spoon onto plates, break up a salmon steak over each plate, and serve.

BROCCOLI BOOST

Broccoli is bursting with nutrition. It contains high levels of both fiber and vitamin C. It is also rich in vitamins A and K, the B vitamins, iron, zinc, and phosphorus. Broccoli is a good source of phytonutrients, which are thought to help reduce the risk of diabetes and heart disease and protect against certain types of cancer.

PER SERVING: 348 CAL | 13.6G FAT | 1.9G SAT FAT | 21.8G CARBS | 6.3G SUGARS | 2.1G SALT | 3.5G FIBER | 35.2G PROTEIN

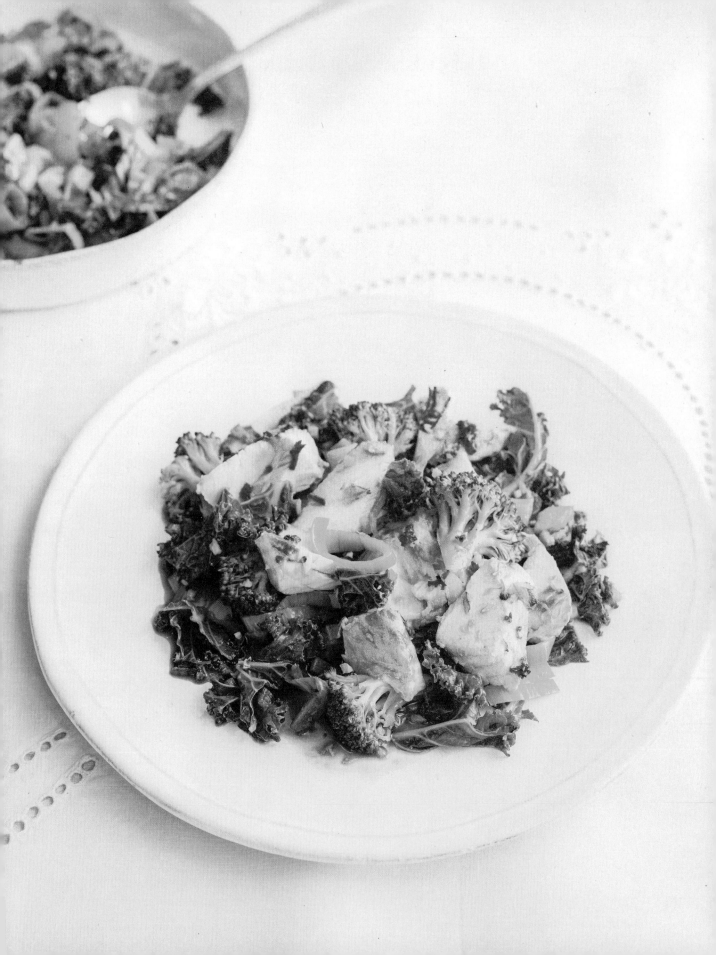

BROILED SALMON WITH MANGO AND LIME SALSA

The refreshing, zingy flavors of mango and lime complement the salmon perfectly in this superfood-packed meal.

SERVES: 4   PREP: 15 MINS   COOK: 10 MINS

2 tablespoons lime juice
1 tablespoon honey
2 tablespoons chopped fresh dill
4 (4-ounce) salmon fillets
salt and pepper, to taste
1 pound new potatoes, boiled, to serve (optional)
salad greens, to serve

MANGO AND LIME SALSA

1 mango, pitted, peeled, and cut into cubes
finely grated zest and juice of 1 lime
2 tablespoons dry unsweetened coconut

1 Preheat the broiler to medium–high and line the broiler rack with aluminum foil.

2 Put the lime juice, honey, and half the dill in a wide bowl and mix well. Season with salt and pepper. Add the salmon and turn to coat in the glaze. Arrange the salmon on the broiler rack, then broil, turning once, for 8–10 minutes, or until browned and the fish flakes easily when pressed with a knife.

3 Meanwhile, to make the salsa, put the mango, lime zest and juice, coconut, and remaining dill in a small bowl and mix well.

4 Serve the salmon, topped with the salsa, with the potatoes, if using, and salad greens on the side.

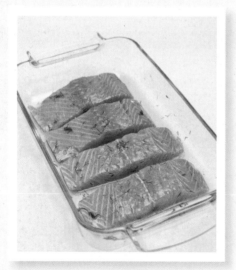

SUPER SALMON

Studies have found that people who eat oily fish, such as salmon, herring, mackerel, or sardines, twice a week are less likely to have heart disease or strokes. It is the omega-3 fatty acids in the fish that help to protect against heart and circulation problems.

PER SERVING: 290 CAL | 17.5G FAT | 6G SAT FAT | 10G CARBS | 9G SUGARS | 0.1G SALT | 3G FIBER | 24G PROTEIN

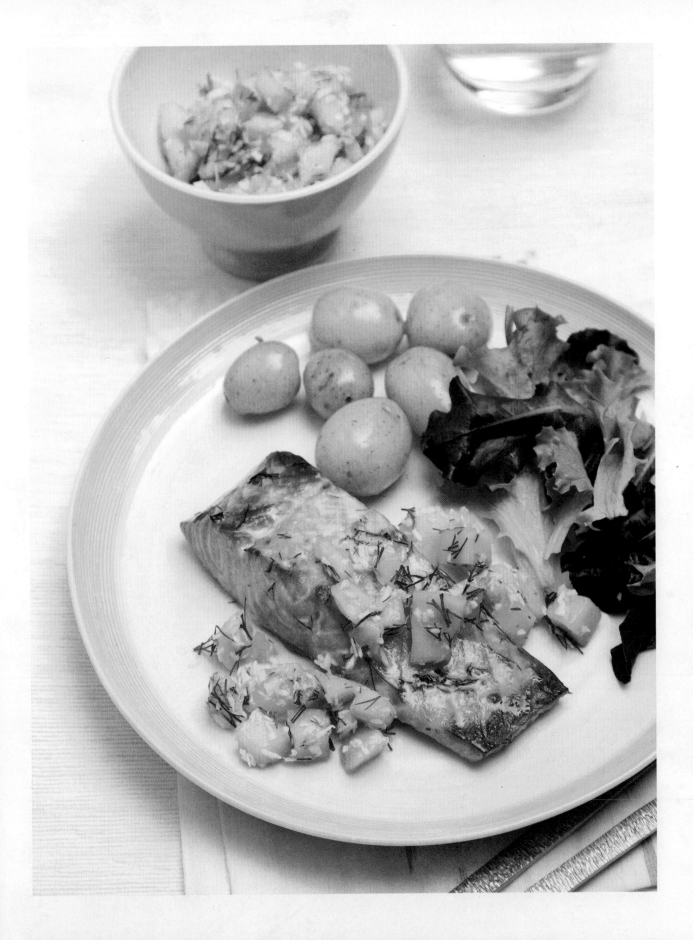

RISOTTO PRIMAVERA

Short-grain brown rice adds a delicious nutty taste to risotto.
It's high in fiber and is believed to help lower cholesterol.

SERVES: 4   PREP: 20 MINS   COOK: 50 MINS

5 cups vegetable stock
1 tablespoon olive oil
1 large leek, thinly sliced, white and green slices kept separate
2 garlic cloves, finely chopped
1/4 cup short-grain brown rice
5 1/2 ounces baby carrots, tops trimmed, halved lengthwise
6 asparagus spears, woody stems removed
1 zucchini, cut into cubes
2 tablespoons butter
3/4 cup finely grated fresh Parmesan cheese
2 1/4 cups mixed baby spinach, watercress, and arugula leaves

1 Bring the stock to a boil in a saucepan.

2 Meanwhile, heat the oil in a large skillet over medium heat. Add the white leek slices and garlic and cook for 3–4 minutes, or until softened but not browned.

3 Stir in the rice and cook for 1 minute. Pour in half the hot stock, bring back to a boil, then cover and simmer for 15 minutes.

4 Add the carrots and half the remaining stock and stir again. Cover and cook for 15 minutes.

5 Add the green leek slices, asparagus, and zucchini, then add a little extra stock. Replace the lid and cook for 5–6 minutes, or until the vegetables and rice are just tender.

6 Remove from the heat, stir in the butter and two-thirds of the cheese, and add a little more stock, if needed. Top with the mixed salad greens, cover with the lid, and warm through for 1–2 minutes, or until the leaves just begin to wilt.

7 Spoon into shallow bowls, sprinkle with the remaining cheese, and serve immediately.

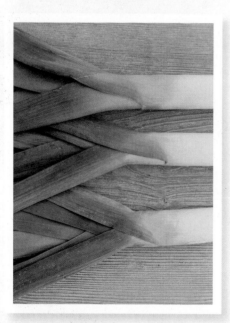

LOVELY LEEKS

Leeks are part of the onion family and contain many antioxidants, minerals, and vitamins, including folic acid, niacin, riboflavin, and thiamin. They are a good source of vitamin A as well as containing vitamins C, E, and K.

PER SERVING: 474 CAL | 17G FAT | 8.1G SAT FAT | 69.4G CARBS | 8.1G SUGARS | 3.8G SALT | 6.4G FIBER | 14.6G PROTEIN

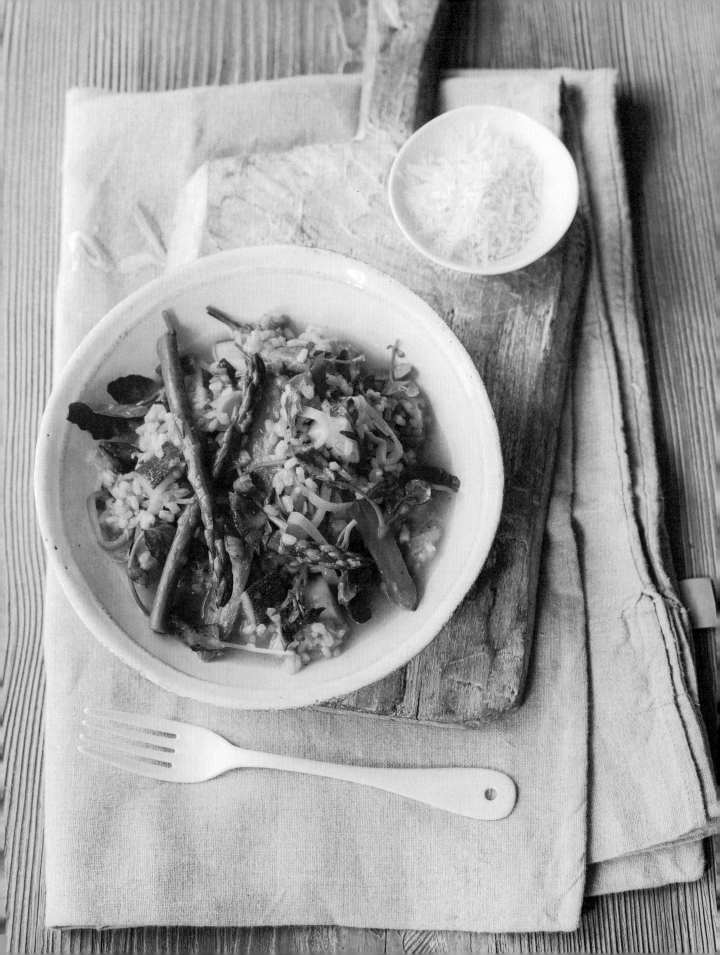

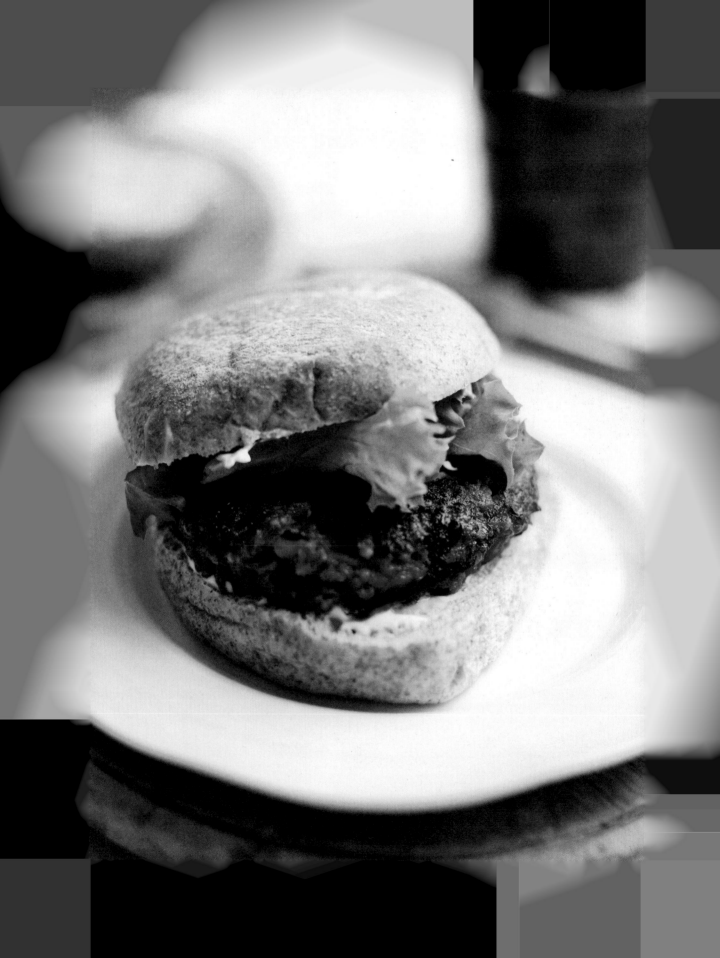

BEET BURGERS
IN BUNS

The sweet, earthy flavor of the vegetables in these wholesome beet-and-millet burgers is delicious with the tangy yogurt sauce.

MAKES: 5 BURGERS
PREP: 30 MINS, PLUS CHILLING   COOK: 35–40 MINS

1/2 cup millet, rinsed and drained
3/4 cup water
2 large raw beets (about 5 1/2 ounces), shredded
1/4 cup shredded carrots
1 zucchini, shredded
1/3 cup finely chopped walnuts
2 tablespoons cider vinegar
2 tablespoons olive oil, plus extra for frying
1 egg, beaten
2 tablespoons cornstarch
salt and pepper, to taste
5 multigrain buns, halved, to serve
lettuce leaves, to serve

YOGURT SAUCE
1 cup plain yogurt
2 garlic cloves, finely chopped

1 Put the millet, water, and a pinch of salt in a small saucepan. Bring to a simmer over medium heat, then reduce the heat to low, cover, and cook for 20–25 minutes, or until tender. Remove from the heat and let stand for 5 minutes, covered.

2 Put the beets, carrots, zucchini, and walnuts into a large bowl. Add the millet, vinegar, oil, 1/2 teaspoon of salt, and 1/2 teaspoon of pepper and mix well. Add the egg and cornstarch, mix again, then cover and chill in the refrigerator for 2 hours.

3 Meanwhile, put the yogurt in a fine-mesh strainer over a bowl and let drain for at least 30 minutes. Stir in the garlic and season with salt and pepper.

4 Spoon the beet mixture into five mounds, then squeeze them into patties using wet hands. Place a ridged grill pan or large skillet over medium heat and coat with olive oil. Add the patties and cook for 10 minutes, or until browned, turning halfway through.

5 Top the bottom of each bun with a spoonful of the yogurt sauce. Place the burgers on top, followed by the lettuce and then the bun lid. Serve immediately.

WOW-FACTOR WALNUTS

Eating a handful of walnuts a day could help protect us against heart disease. Scientists have found that they may improve cholesterol levels and blood vessel flexibility.

PER BURGER: 486 CAL | 17.2G FAT | 3G SAT FAT | 70.5G CARBS | 15G SUGARS | 2G SALT | 8.1G FIBER | 16G PROTEIN

STUFFED RED PEPPERS

A little ground beef goes a long way in this rustic-style dish that's packed with nutritious beans and lentils.

SERVES: 4   PREP: 20 MINS   COOK: 1 HOUR

4 large red bell peppers, stems left on, halved lengthwise and seeded
1 tablespoon olive oil
1 red onion, finely chopped
1 pound ground round or ground sirloin beef
2 garlic cloves, finely chopped
¼ teaspoon smoked hot paprika or chili powder
1 teaspoon ground cumin
1 (15-ounce) can chickpeas, drained
2 cups cooked or drained and rinsed canned green lentils
1 (14½-ounce) can diced tomatoes
½ cup beef stock
salt and pepper, to taste
¾ cup fat-free Greek-style plain yogurt (optional)
¼ cup coarsely chopped fresh mint
¼ cup coarsely chopped fresh flat-leaf parsley

1   Preheat the oven to 350°F. Arrange the bell peppers cut-side up in a roasting pan.

2   Heat the oil in a skillet over medium heat. Add the red onion, ground beef, and garlic and cook, stirring and breaking up the meat, for 5 minutes, or until evenly browned.

3   Stir in the paprika and cumin, then the chickpeas, lentils, tomatoes, and stock. Season with salt and pepper, then increase the heat to high and bring to a boil. Remove from the heat.

4   Spoon the meat mixture into the bell peppers, cover the dish with aluminum foil, then bake for 50 minutes, or until the bell peppers are tender and the meat is cooked.

5   Remove the foil, top each bell pepper with a large spoonful of yogurt, if using, then sprinkle generously with the mint and parsley and serve immediately.

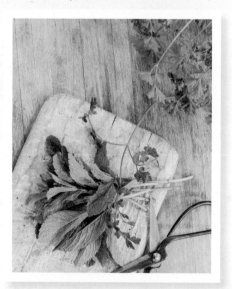

FRAGRANT MINT

Mint is rich in antioxidants and phytonutrients that are thought to be good for the stomach. It has anti-inflammatory properties, so is believed to be beneficial for the skin, too. Some health experts also say it relieves headaches and menstrual cramps.

PER SERVING: 466 CAL | 16.2G FAT | 5G SAT FAT | 40.8G CARBS | 11.9G SUGARS | 1.3G SALT | 9.1G FIBER | 36G PROTEIN

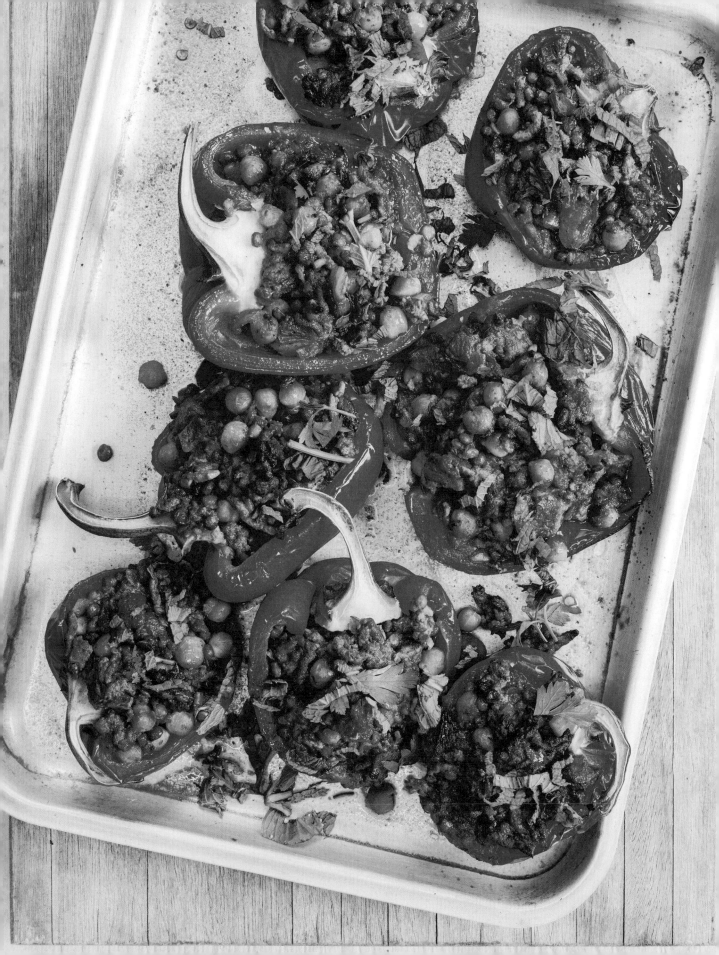

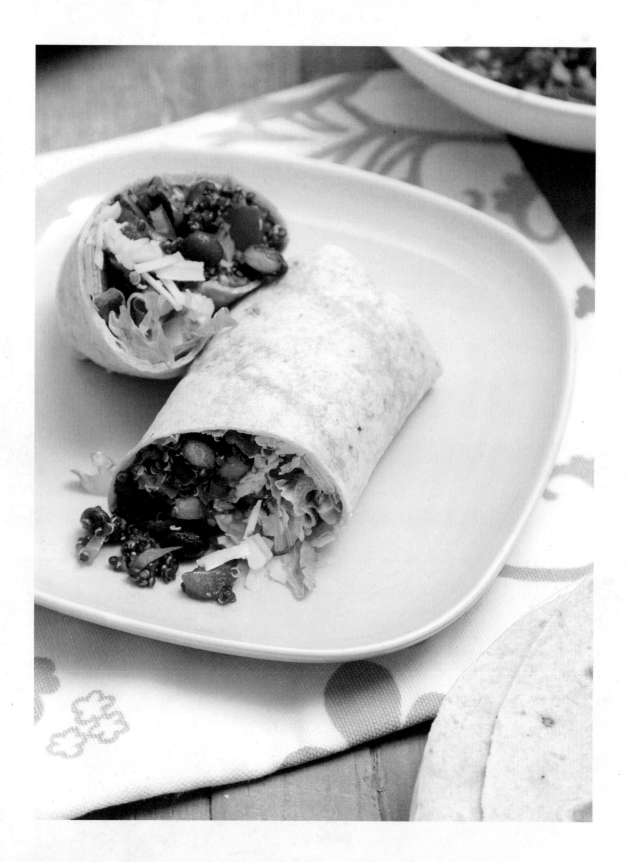

BLACK BEAN AND QUINOA BURRITOS

*This Mexican-American treat is filling enough for a main meal,
but is equally good served cold or packed into a lunch bag.*

MAKES: 8 BURRITOS
PREP: 30 MINS   COOK: 20 MINS, PLUS STANDING

1/3 cup red quinoa, rinsed
2/3 cup water
2 tablespoons vegetable oil
1 red onion, coarsely chopped
1 green chile, seeded and finely chopped
1 small red bell pepper, seeded and cut into cubes
1 (15-ounce) can black beans, drained and rinsed
juice of 1 lime
1/3 cup coarsely chopped fresh cilantro
2 tomatoes
8 corn tortillas, warmed
1 cup shredded cheddar cheese
1 1/2 cups shredded romaine lettuce
salt and pepper, to taste

1 Put the quinoa, water, and a pinch of salt into a small saucepan. Bring to a boil, then cover and simmer over a low heat for 15 minutes, or according to package directions. Remove from the heat, but keep the pan covered for 5 minutes to let the grains swell. Fluff up with a fork.

2 Heat the oil in a skillet over medium heat. Add half the red onion, half the green chile, and half the red bell pepper and cook until softened. Add the beans, cooked quinoa, half the lime juice, and half the cilantro and cook for 3–4 minutes. Season with salt and pepper.

3 Halve the tomatoes and scoop out the seeds. Add the seeds to the bean mixture. Finely chop the flesh and transfer it to a bowl. Add the remaining red onion, green chile, red bell pepper, lime juice, and cilantro to the bowl, season with salt and stir well.

4 Put 1/3 cup of the bean mixture on top of each tortilla. Sprinkle with the tomato salsa, cheese, and lettuce. Fold the end and sides of the tortillas over the filling, roll up, and serve.

RAINBOW VEG

Try to broaden the types and colors of the vegetables you eat: the brighter the better for the maximum range of health-protecting antioxidants and phytochemicals in your diet.

PER BURRITO: 270 CAL | 10.4G FAT | 3.9G SAT FAT | 36.7G CARBS | 1.8G SUGARS | 0.7G SALT | 5.2G FIBER | 9.3G PROTEIN

RAW SPROUTS AND SEEDS SUPERSALAD

Sprouting seeds are bursting with nutrients and low in calories, making this superfood dish superlight as well as superhealthy.

SERVES: 6   PREP: 15 MINS

8 ounces mixed seed and bean sprouts, such as alfalfa, mung beans, soybeans, aduki beans, chickpeas, and radish seeds
3 tablespoons pumpkin seeds
3 tablespoons sunflower seeds
3 tablespoons sesame seeds
1 crisp, sweet apple, cored and coarsely chopped
1/2 cup coarsely chopped dried apricots
finely grated zest and juice of 1 unwaxed lemon
1/2 cup coarsely chopped walnuts
2 tablespoons walnut oil

1   Put the seed and bean sprouts, pumpkin seeds, sunflower seeds, and sesame seeds into a large bowl. Stir in the apple and dried apricots, lemon zest, and walnuts.

2   To make the dressing, put the lemon juice and the oil in a small bowl and mix together with a fork.

3   Stir the dressing into the salad, then serve immediately.

SPROUTING SEEDS

Sprouting seeds are a quick and easy way of filling up with nutrients. Studies show they contain high levels of the B vitamins, as well as vitamins A, C, and E.

PER SERVING: 228 CAL | 17.8G FAT | 1.9G SAT FAT | 15G CARBS | 8.7G SUGARS | TRACE SALT | 4G FIBER | 6.7G PROTEIN

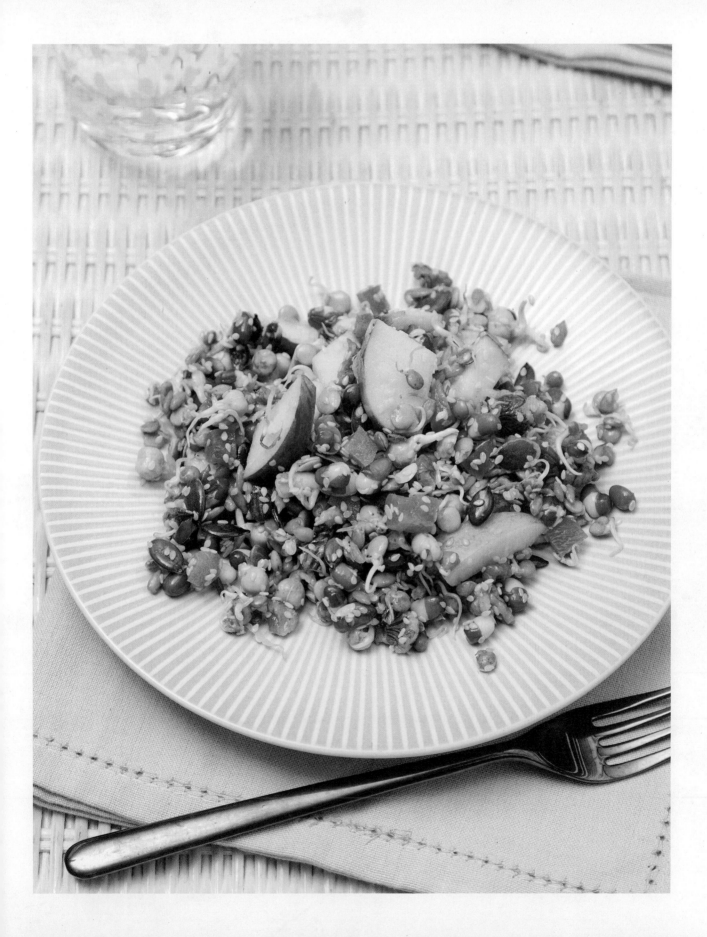

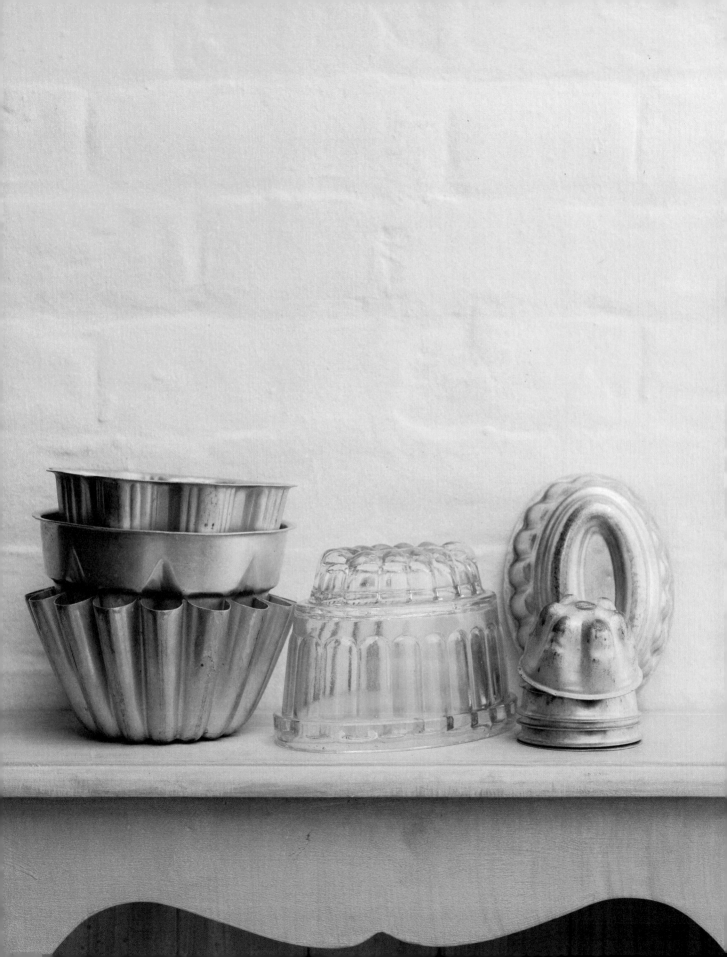

DESSERTS AND BAKING

Chocolate, cinnamon, and vanilla custard desserts — 102

Chocolate, fruit, and nut bark — 104

Skinny banana split sundaes — 106

Warm walnut and orange cake — 108

Summer berry sponge cakes — 110

Creamy coconut and mango quinoa — 112

Broiled peaches and nectarines — 114

Cranberry and raspberry gelatin — 116

Strawberries with balsamic vinegar — 119

Green tea fruit salad — 120

Raspberry and watermelon sorbet — 122

Fruit cocktail ice pops — 124

CHOCOLATE, CINNAMON, AND VANILLA CUSTARD DESSERTS

Rich, dark, and smooth, these easy-to-make desserts not only look fabulous but will also satisfy any chocolate craving.

MAKES: 6 DESSERTS

PREP: 20 MINS COOK: 50 MINS CHILL: 5 HOURS

2 cups low-fat milk
7 ounces semisweet chocolate (at least 65 percent cocoa solids), broken into pieces, plus 1 tablespoon finely grated semisweet chocolate to decorate
1 teaspoon vanilla extract
1/4 teaspoon ground cinnamon
1/4 cup honey
2 eggs, plus 2 egg yolks
1/3 cup fat-free Greek-style plain yogurt, to decorate

1 Preheat the oven to 300°F. Pour the milk into a heavy-based saucepan, bring just to a boil, then remove from the heat and stir in the chocolate pieces, vanilla extract, ground cinnamon, and 3 tablespoons of honey. Set aside for 5 minutes, or until the chocolate has melted. Stir until the milk is an even dark chocolate color.

2 Put the eggs and egg yolks into a large bowl and beat lightly with a fork. Gradually pour in the warm chocolate milk, beating all the time with a wooden spoon, until smooth. Strain back into the saucepan through a strainer, then press any remaining chocolate through the strainer using the back of the spoon.

3 Put six 3/4-cup ovenproof teacups or ramekins (ceramic dishes) into a roasting pan. Fill the cups with the chocolate mixture, then pour hot water into the roasting pan to reach halfway up the cups. Cover the cups with aluminum foil, then bake for 40–45 minutes, or until the custards are just set, with a slight wobble in the center.

4 Using oven mitts, lift the cups out of the roasting pan and let cool, then cover with plastic wrap and chill in the refrigerator for 4–5 hours.

5 Place the cups on a serving plate, remove the plastic wrap, and top each with a spoonful of yogurt, a drizzle of the remaining honey, and a little grated chocolate.

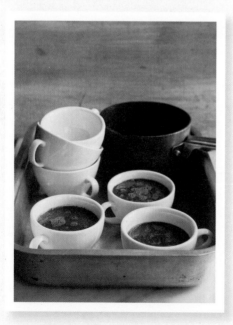

DARK CHOCOLATE IS GOOD FOR YOU!

Research shows that dark chocolate is packed with antioxidants and may help lower blood pressure, but it must have 65 percent or ideally more cocoa content. The darker it is, the less fat and sugar it will probably contain.

PER CUP: 343 CAL | 19.5G FAT | 10.6G SAT FAT | 32.3G CARBS | 24.5G SUGARS | 0.2G SALT | 3.8G FIBER | 10G PROTEIN

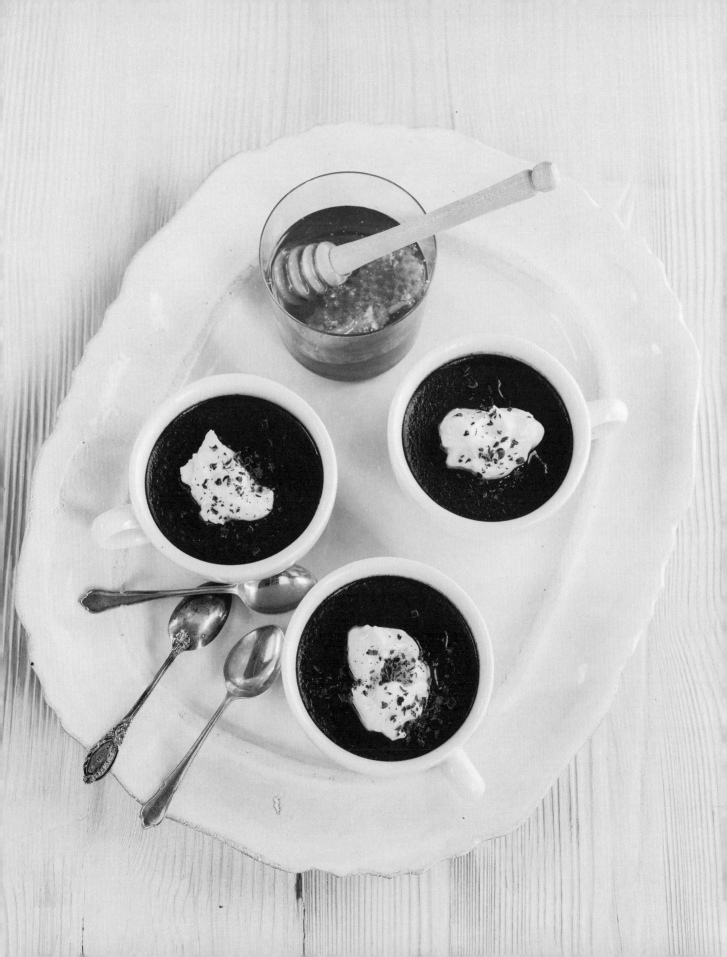

CHOCOLATE, FRUIT, AND NUT BARK

Hazelnuts and chocolate make this snack a superfood treat that's perfect for wrapping in parchment paper and packing into your lunch bag.

MAKES: 16 PIECES

PREP: 15 MINS   COOK: 4 MINS   CHILL: 1 HOUR

1/2 cup dried cherries
1/2 cup coarsely chopped hazelnuts
12 ounces bittersweet chocolate (at least
70 percent cocoa solids), broken into pieces
1/2 cup crispy rice cereal

1 Line an 11 x 9-inch baking pan with parchment paper.

2 Put the dried cherries and hazelnuts into a small bowl and mix well.

3 Put the chocolate in a heatproof bowl set over a saucepan of gently simmering water, making sure the bowl doesn't touch the water, and heat until melted. Remove from the heat and stir in the rice cereal.

4 Pour the chocolate mixture into the prepared pan and smooth it into a thin layer, using a spatula. Immediately sprinkle the dried cherries and hazelnuts over the chocolate mixture, then press them into it with the palm of your hand. Cover with plastic wrap and chill in the refrigerator for 1 hour, or until set.

5 Break into 16 pieces and serve at room temperature.

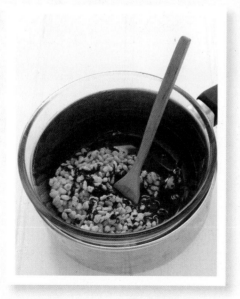

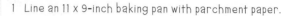

GO HAZELNUTS!

Hazelnuts are rich in vitamin E and contain protein and vitamin A. They are loaded with minerals, too, especially manganese, selenium, and zinc.

PER PIECE: 171 CAL | 11.4G FAT | 5.5G SAT FAT | 15G CARBS | 7.5G SUGARS | TRACE SALT | 3.8G FIBER | 2.4G PROTEIN

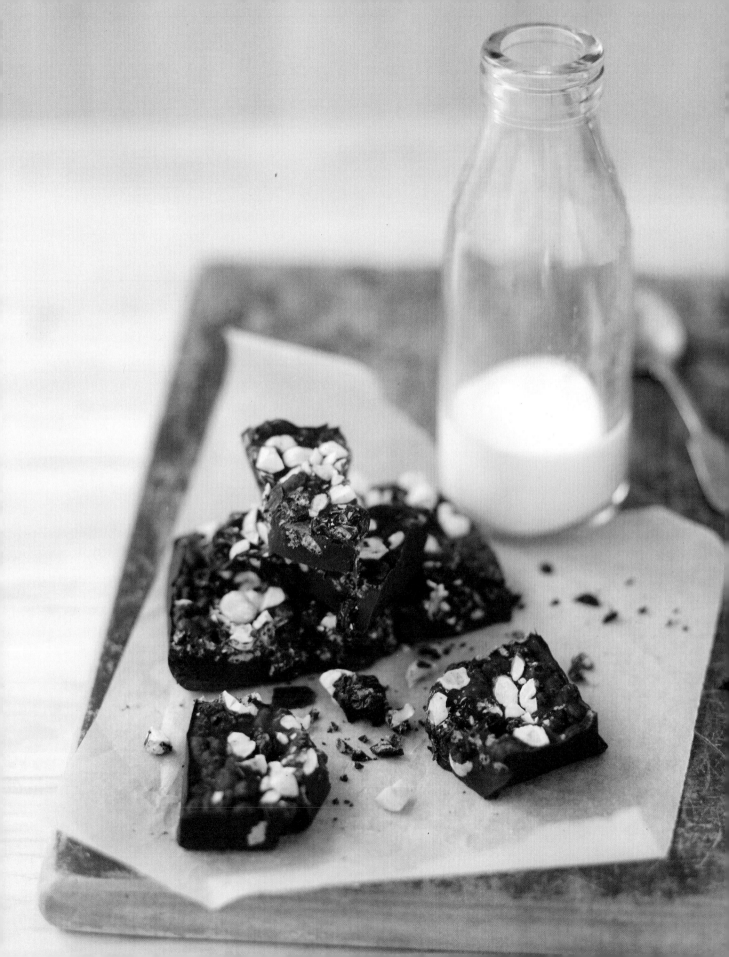

SKINNY BANANA SPLIT SUNDAES

Keep this twist on a traditional sundae in the freezer, then make the chocolate sauce just before serving, for a superfood-packed standby dessert everyone will love.

SERVES: 2
PREP: 10 MINS   COOK: 6 MINS   FREEZE: 3 HOURS

2 small bananas, peeled and coarsely chopped
6 unblanched almonds, coarsely chopped

CHOCOLATE SAUCE
2 tablespoons packed light brown sugar
3 tablespoons unsweetened cocoa powder
1/3 cup plus 1 tablespoon low-fat milk
1 ounce bittersweet chocolate (at least 70 percent cocoa solids), broken into pieces
1/2 teaspoon vanilla extract

1 Put the bananas into a plastic container and freeze for 2 hours. Transfer to a food processor and process until smooth and creamy. Return to the container, replace the lid, and freeze for 1 hour, or until firm.

2 To make the chocolate sauce, put the sugar, cocoa powder, and milk into a small saucepan and bring to a simmer over medium heat. Reduce the heat to low and cook, stirring constantly, for 1 minute, or until the sugar and cocoa powder have dissolved.

3 Remove from the heat, then stir in the chocolate until it has melted. Stir in the vanilla extract. Let cool slightly.

4 Place a skillet over high heat. Add the almonds, cover, and dry-fry for 3–4 minutes, or until toasted.

5 Scoop the banana puree into two glasses or bowls, drizzle with the warm chocolate sauce, and sprinkle with the almonds.

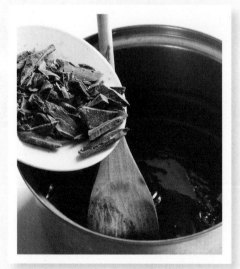

AMAZING ALMONDS

Almonds are a rich source of calcium, protein, essential fats, the B vitamins, and vitamin E. They also contain iron, potassium, and magnesium, as well as copper, which is needed in red blood cell production and so can help prevent anemia.

PER SERVING: 311 CAL | 11.3G FAT | 5.1G SAT FAT | 52.9G CARBS | 33.7G SUGARS | TRACE SALT | 7.5G FIBER | 6.4G PROTEIN

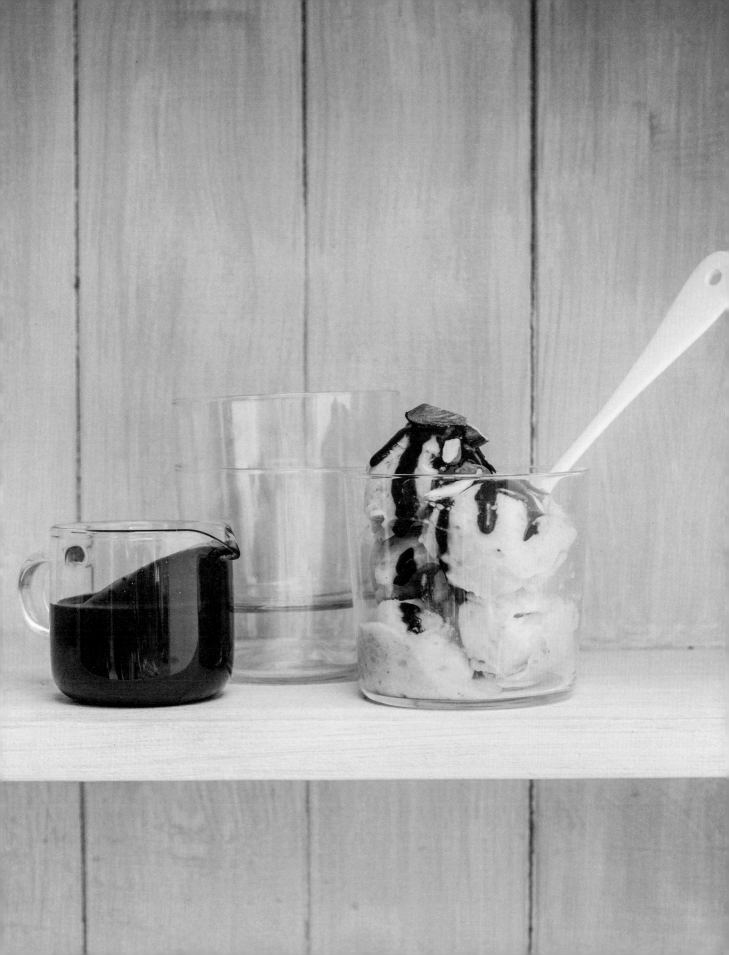

WARM WALNUT AND ORANGE CAKE

A Middle Eastern-inspired cake that is gluten-free and packed with energy-boosting nuts. The whole cooked orange gives it a tangy, high-fiber citrus hit.

MAKES: 10 SLICES   PREP: 25 MINS   COOK: 2¼ HOURS

3 large whole oranges

1 cup dried apricots

2/3 cup coarsely chopped walnuts, plus 12 halves to decorate

3/4 cup unblanched almonds, coarsely chopped, plus 6 to decorate

1/2 cup Brazil nuts, coarsely chopped, plus 12 to decorate

4 eggs

1 cup superfine or granulated sugar

1/2 cup light olive oil, plus extra to grease

1/2 cup brown rice flour

2 teaspoons gluten-free baking powder

1 cup fat-free Greek-style plain yogurt, to serve

BRILLIANT BRAZIL NUTS

Brazil nuts are a good source of the mineral selenium, which we need to produce the active thyroid hormone, and which helps boost your immune system. They are also rich in protein and fiber.

1   Put one orange in a small saucepan, just cover with water, then bring to a boil, cover, and simmer for 45 minutes. Add the dried apricots, replace the lid, and cook for 15 minutes, or until the orange is tender when pierced with a knife. Drain the fruits, reserving the cooking water, and let cool.

2   Preheat the oven to 325°F. Lightly brush a 9½-inch round springform cake pan with a little oil. Put the measured walnuts, almonds, and Brazil nuts into a food processor and process until finely ground. Transfer to a large mixing bowl.

3   Coarsely chop the cooked orange, discard any seeds, then put it and the apricots in a food processor and process into a coarse puree. Add the eggs, 3/4 cup of sugar and all the oil, and process again until smooth.

4   Spoon the brown rice flour and baking powder into the ground nuts and mix well. Transfer to the food processor and process briefly until smooth. Pour the cake batter into the prepared pan, spread it level with a spatula, and decorate with the walnut halves, whole almonds, and whole Brazil nuts.

5   Bake for 1–1¼ hours, or until browned, slightly cracked on top, and a toothpick inserted into the center comes out clean. Check after 40 minutes and loosely cover the top with aluminum foil if the nut decoration is browning too quickly.

6   Cut the peel and pith away from the remaining oranges with a small serrated knife. Cut between the membranes to release the segments. Measure 1/2 cup of the reserved orange cooking water, making it up with extra water, if needed, and pour it into a small saucepan. Add the remaining sugar and cook over low heat until the sugar has dissolved. Increase the heat to high and boil for 3 minutes, or until you have a syrup. Add the orange segments and let cool.

7   Loosen the edge of the cake with a blunt knife and turn out onto a wire rack. Let cool slightly, then cut into wedges and serve warm, with the oranges in syrup and spoonfuls of the Greek yogurt.

PER SLICE: 517 CAL | 33.7G FAT | 5.3G SAT FAT | 47.4G CARBS | 34.6G SUGARS | 0.8G SALT | 5.2G FIBER | 11.9G PROTEIN

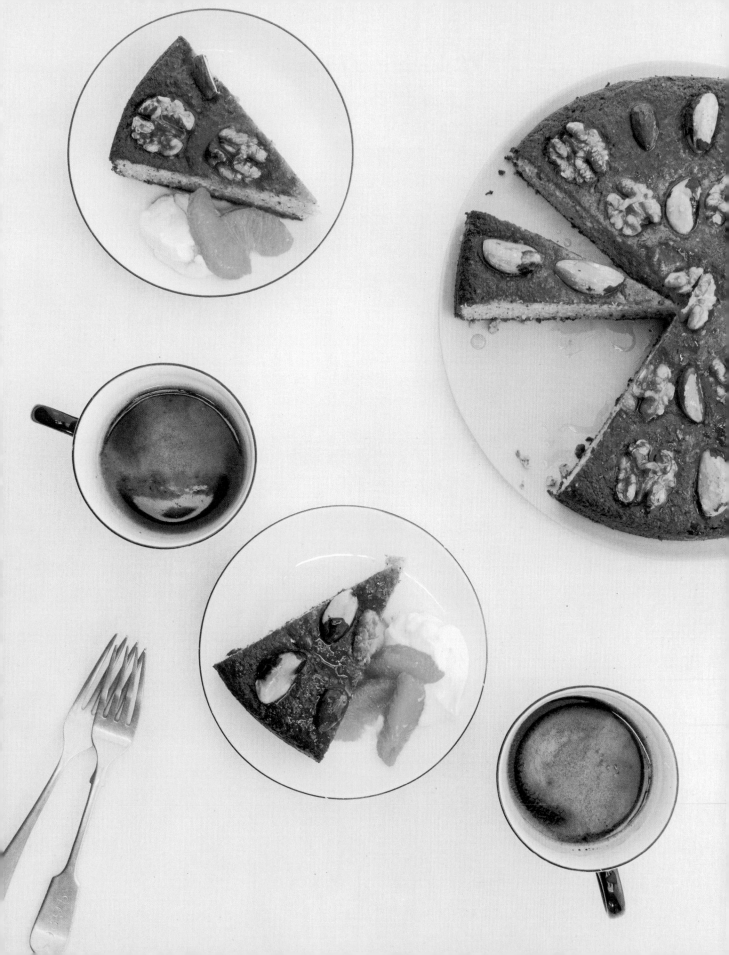

SUMMER BERRY SPONGE CAKES

These light sponge cakes are made without butter and filled with fat-free Greek yogurt for a sweet treat that doesn't look or taste low calorie.

MAKES: 6 CAKES   PREP: 25 MINS   COOK: 15 MINS

vegetable oil, to grease
3 eggs
1/3 cup superfine or granulated sugar
1/2 teaspoon vanilla extract
1/2 cup brown rice flour
1 cup fat-free Greek-style natural yogurt
3 1/2 cups mixed berries, such as raspberries, blueberries, and hulled and sliced strawberries
1 tablespoon confectioners' sugar

1 Preheat the oven to 350°F. Brush six 3/4-cup tube pans with a little oil and put them on a baking sheet.

2 Put the eggs, superfine sugar, and vanilla extract into a large bowl and beat with an electric handheld mixer for 5 minutes, or until the mixture is thick and leaves a trail when the beaters are lifted.

3 Sift the flour over the egg mixture, then gently fold it in with a large metal spoon. Spoon the batter into the pans and ease it into an even layer, being careful not to knock out any air.

4 Bake for 12–15 minutes, or until the cakes are risen and golden brown and beginning to shrink away from the edges of the pans.

5 Let cool for 5 minutes. Loosen the edges of the cakes with a blunt knife and turn them out onto a wire rack. Let cool completely.

6 Put the cakes on serving plates, spoon the yogurt into the center, then pile the fruits on top. Sift confectioners' sugar over the fruit and cakes and serve.

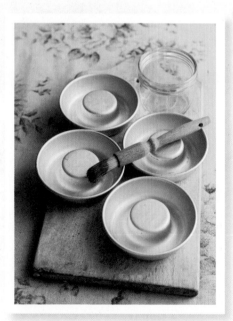

RASPBERRY GOODNESS

Raspberries are bursting with vitamin C and contain powerful antioxidants that are thought to help boost the immune system and protect us from cancers. They are also rich in the B vitamins and vitamin K.

PER CAKE: 219 CAL | 4.5G FAT | 1G SAT FAT | 36.3G CARBS | 22.6G SUGARS | 0.1G SALT | 2.8G FIBER | 9.3G PROTEIN

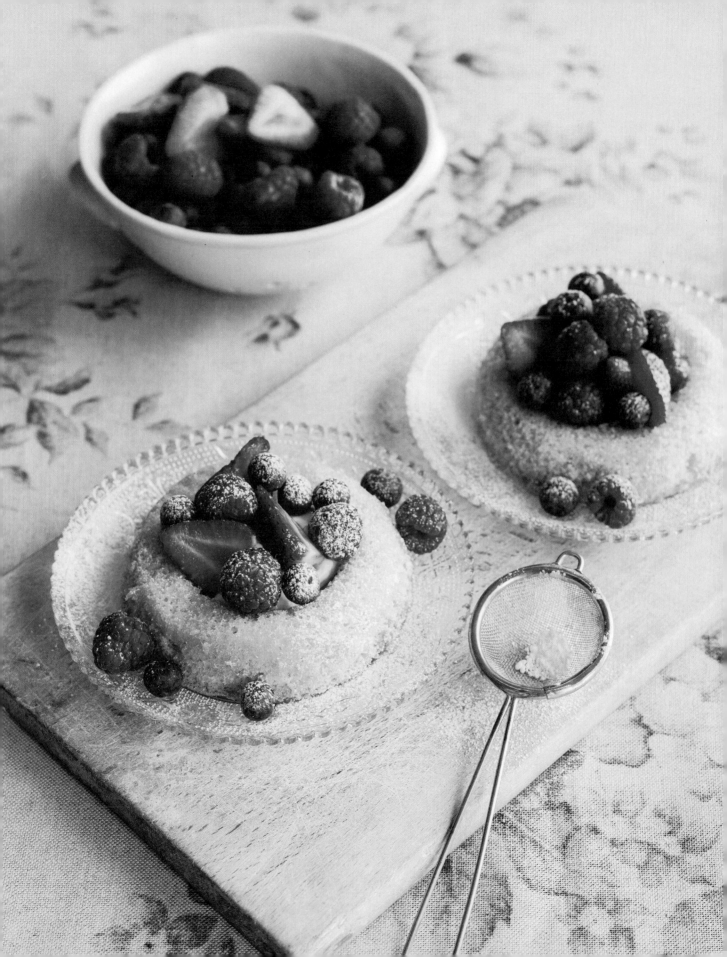

CREAMY COCONUT AND MANGO QUINOA

*Forget white rice — this healthy take on rice pudding
is made with nutrient-dense quinoa.*

SERVES: 4
PREP: 15 MINS, PLUS STANDING   COOK: 20 MINS

1¼ cups coconut milk
⅔ cup quinoa, rinsed
1 large mango, pitted, peeled, and coarsely chopped
⅓ cup superfine or granulated sugar
juice of 1 large lime
1½-inch piece fresh ginger, peeled and cut into chunks
⅔ cup blueberries
¼ cup toasted dry coconut shavings

1 Put the coconut milk and quinoa into a small saucepan and bring to a boil over medium heat. Reduce the heat to low, cover, and simmer for 10–15 minutes, or according to the package directions, until most of the liquid has evaporated. Remove from the heat and set aside for 7 minutes to let the grains swell. Fluff up with a fork, transfer to a bowl, and let cool.

2 Meanwhile, put the mango, sugar, and lime juice into a food processor. Squeeze the ginger through a garlic press and add the juice to the food processor. Process for 30 seconds, or until you have a smooth puree.

3 Mix the mango puree into the cooled quinoa, then cover and let stand for 30 minutes.

4 Spoon the mixture into four bowls and sprinkle with the blueberries and coconut shavings. Serve immediately.

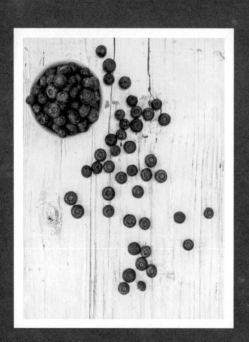

BRILLIANT BLUEBERRIES

Blueberries have a high concentration of antioxidants, which are thought to help prevent heart disease and even cancer. They are rich in manganese, fiber, which helps keep your cholesterol low, and vitamin C for immunity.

PER SERVING: 408 CAL | 16.7G FAT | 13.2G SAT FAT | 60.8G CARBS | 37.2G SUGARS | TRACE SALT | 5G FIBER | 6.5G PROTEIN

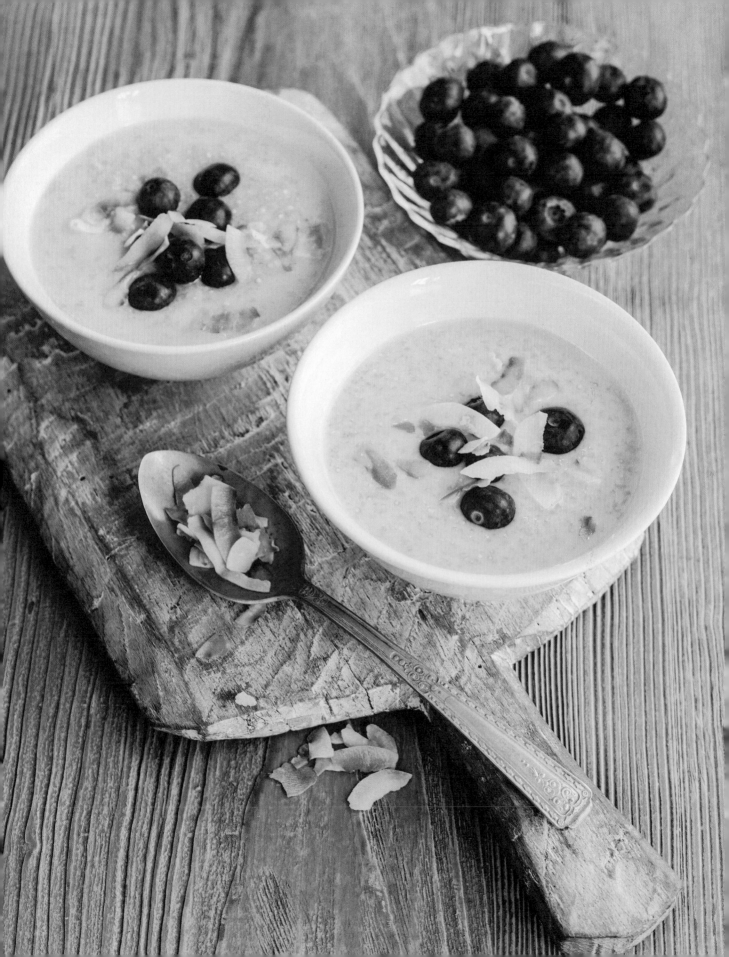

BROILED PEACHES AND NECTARINES

When you need a glamorous dessert but you're in a rush, this low-fat treat bursting with fresh fruit is just the thing.

SERVES: 6   PREP: 10 MINS   COOK: 5 MINS

1¹/2 cups low-fat ricotta cheese
2 teaspoons finely grated orange zest
3 peaches, pitted and quartered
3 nectarines, pitted and quartered
3 plums or apricots, pitted and quartered
2 tablespoons honey, ideally orange blossom
2 tablespoons slivered almonds

1 Preheat the broiler to medium–high. Line the broiler rack with aluminum foil.

2 Put the ricotta and orange zest in a bowl and stir well.

3 Lay all the fruit in a single layer on the foil-lined broiler rack. Broil the fruit, turning halfway, for 5 minutes, or until softened and beginning to caramelize.

4 Spoon the ricotta into six glasses. Top each with some broiled fruit, drizzle with the honey, and sprinkle with the slivered almonds. Serve immediately.

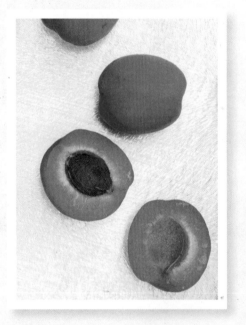

REACH FOR APRICOTS

Apricots are rich in beta-carotene, which is important for vision, and vitamin C. They are also a good source of fiber and minerals, such as potassium and manganese.

PER SERVING: 202 CAL | 7.1G FAT | 3.2G SAT FAT | 28.1G CARBS | 21.2G SUGARS | 0.2G SALT | 3.2G FIBER | 9.5G PROTEIN

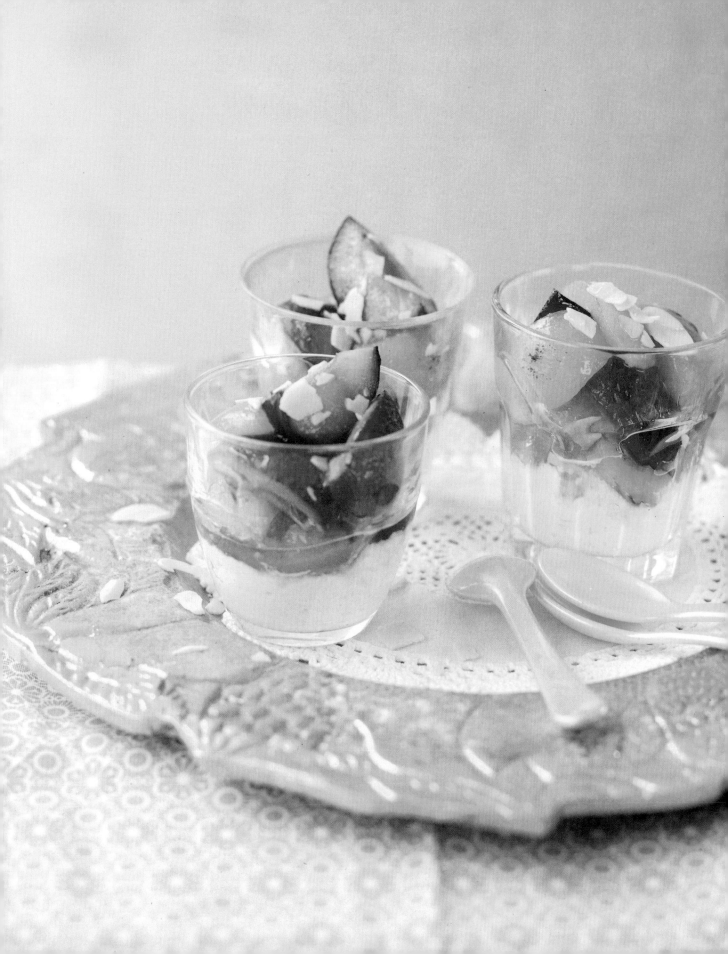

CRANBERRY AND RASPBERRY GELATIN

Beloved of children's parties, gelatin is popular with all ages—and it's virtually fat free. This cranberry gelatin has a delicious grown-up flavor and beautiful color.

SERVES: 6   PREP: 15 MINS
COOK: 15 MINS   CHILL AND FREEZE: 7 1/4 HOURS

3 1/2 cups frozen cranberries
1/3 cup superfine or granulated sugar
2 1/2 cups water, plus extra for the gelatin
4 gelatin sheets
1 1/2 cups frozen raspberries, plus a few extra to serve

1 Put the frozen cranberries, sugar, and 1 cup of water into a saucepan, cover, and cook over medium heat for 10–15 minutes, or until soft. Let cool.

2 Meanwhile, put the gelatin sheets in a shallow dish, cover with cold water, and let soften for 5 minutes.

3 Pour the cranberries and their cooking liquid into a food processor and process to a puree. Push the puree through a fine-mesh strainer back into the saucepan, then stir in the remaining water and warm over low heat.

4 Drain the gelatin sheets, add to the warm cranberry mixture, and stir until the gelatin has dissolved. Let cool.

5 Arrange a ring of frozen raspberries in the bottom of a 1 1/4-quart gelatin mold, then spoon a little of the cranberry mixture over the top. Freeze for 15–20 minutes, or until set.

6 Pour half the remaining cranberry mixture into the mold, sprinkle with half the remaining raspberries, then chill in the refrigerator for 1 hour, or until just set. Pour the remaining cranberry mixture over the raspberries and sprinkle with the remaining raspberries. Chill in the refrigerator for 4–6 hours, or until set firm.

7 Dip the mold into a bowl of hot water, count to ten, then lift it out. Invert the mold onto a plate, then—holding the mold and the plate tightly—jerk to release the gelatin. Remove the mold and serve.

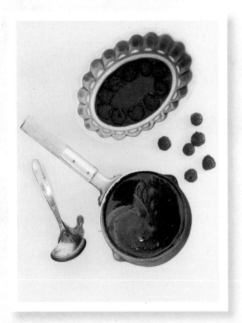

CRANBERRY PROTECTION

These bright red, tart-tasting berries are rich in vitamins C and A and potassium. Their phytochemicals may help prevent and aid recovery from cystitis and other urinary tract infections.

PER SERVING: 106 CAL | 0.3G FAT | TRACE SAT FAT | 25.3G CARBS | 18G SUGARS | TRACE SALT | 4.8G FIBER | 2.4G PROTEIN

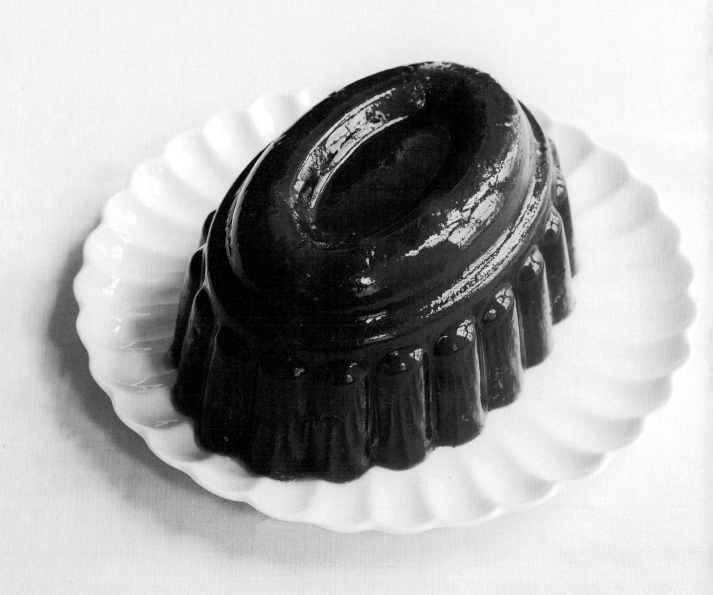

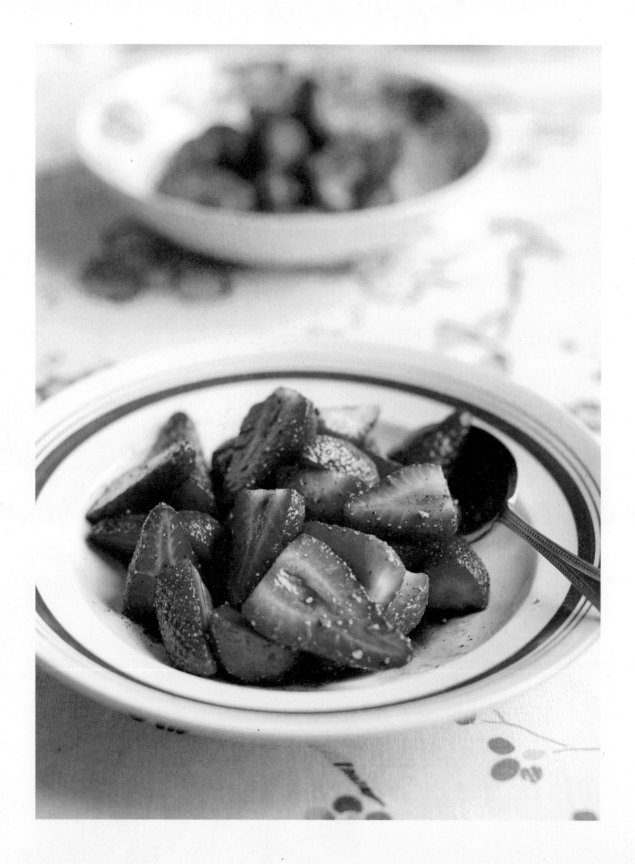

STRAWBERRIES WITH BALSAMIC VINEGAR

Proving simplicity really can be best, this summer dessert combines sweetness, spice, and acidity in the most delicious way. Be sure to use only the best strawberries.

SERVES: 4   PREP: 5 MINS   STAND: 3 HOURS

2 tablespoons superfine or granulated sugar
1 tablespoon balsamic vinegar
2 1/2 cups hulled and halved strawberries
pepper, to taste

1   Put the sugar and vinegar in a nonmetallic bowl and stir. Add the strawberries and stir well. Let stand for at least 1 hour, but for no more than 3 hours.

2   Stir again, then add extra sugar or vinegar, if desired.

3   Grind some pepper over the top of the strawberries and serve immediately.

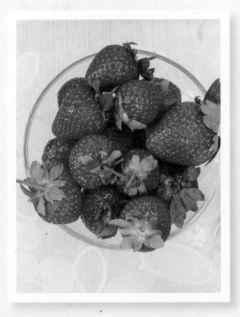

SENSATIONAL STRAWBERRIES

Strawberries contain a lot of vitamin C and are relatively high in fiber. They are also an excellent source of the mineral manganese, which is good for bone health.

PER SERVING: 64 CAL | 0.3G FAT | TRACE SAT FAT | 15.7G CARBS | 12.5G SUGARS | TRACE SALT | 2.2G FIBER | 0.7G PROTEIN

GREEN TEA FRUIT SALAD

The delicate and refreshing taste of green tea works well mixed with chopped fresh mint and a hint of honey in a syrup for a fruit salad.

SERVES: 4   PREP: 15 MINS   CHILL: 1 HOUR

2 teaspoons green tea
1 cup boiling water
1 tablespoon honey
1/2 small watermelon, seeded, peeled, and cut into cubes
1 large mango, pitted, peeled, and cut into cubes
1 papaya, seeded, peeled, and cut into cubes
2 pears, peeled, cored, and cut into cubes
2 kiwis, peeled and cut into cubes
2 tablespoons coarsely chopped fresh mint
seeds of 1/2 pomegranate
2 tablespoons coarsely chopped pistachio nuts

1 Put the tea into a teapot or saucepan, pour boiling water over the leaves, and let brew for 3–4 minutes. Strain into a small bowl, stir in the honey, and let cool.

2 Put the watermelon, mango, and papaya into a large serving bowl, then add the pears, kiwis, and mint. Pour the cooled green tea over the fruits and stir gently.

3 Cover the fruit salad with plastic wrap and chill in the refrigerator for 1 hour. Stir gently to mix the tea through the fruits.

4 Spoon the fruit salad into four bowls and serve sprinkled with the pomegranate seeds and pistachio nuts.

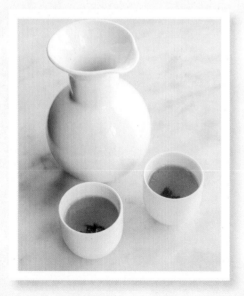

GO FOR GREEN TEA

Green tea is used in traditional Chinese medicine. It contains antioxidants, and is thought to have antibacterial and antiviral properties.

PER SERVING: 313 CAL | 4.8G FAT | 0.6G SAT FAT | 70.8G CARBS | 54G SUGARS | TRACE SALT | 10G FIBER | 5.2G PROTEIN

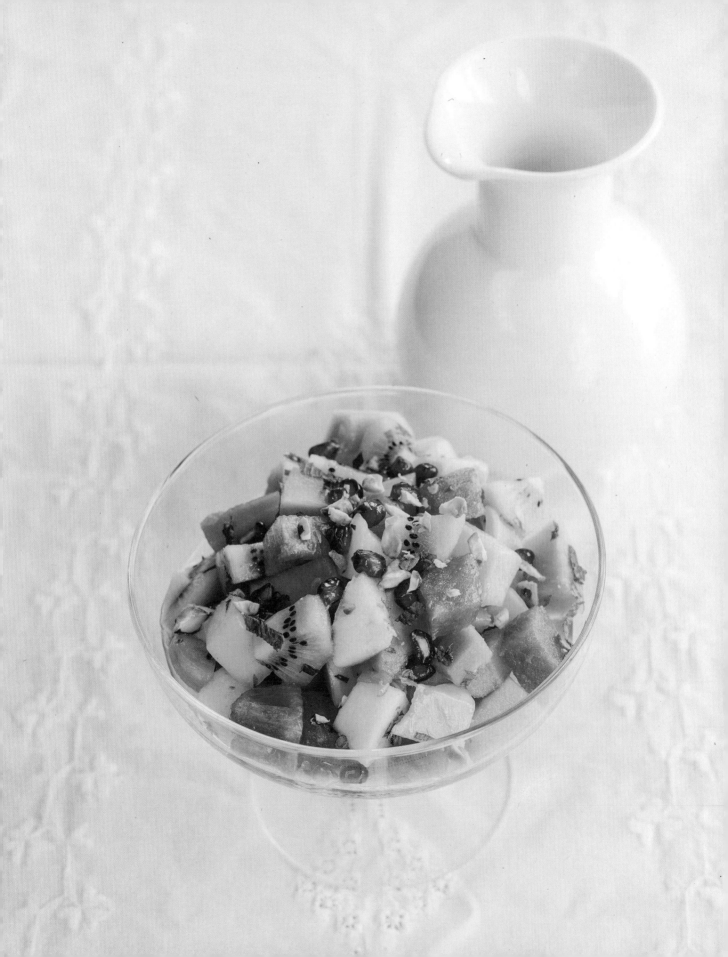

RASPBERRY AND WATERMELON SORBET

Wonderfully refreshing on a hot day, or soothing after a spicy meal,
this healthy and easy-to-make dessert is great to have tucked away in the freezer.

SERVES: 4   PREP: 20 MINS
COOK: 4 MINS   FREEZE: 8 HOURS

2/3 cup superfine or granulated sugar
2/3 cup cold water
finely grated zest and juice of 1 lime
1 3/4 cups raspberries
1 small watermelon, seeded, peeled, and
cut into chunks
1 egg white

1 Put the sugar, water, and lime zest into a small saucepan and cook over low heat, stirring, until the sugar has dissolved. Increase the heat to high until the mixture comes to a boil, then reduce to medium and simmer for 3–4 minutes. Let cool completely.

2 Put the raspberries and watermelon into a food processor in batches and process to a puree, then press through a strainer into a bowl to remove any remaining seeds.

3 Transfer the puree to a loaf pan, pour in the lime syrup through a strainer, then stir in the lime juice. Freeze for 3–4 hours, or until the sorbet is beginning to freeze around the edges but the center is still mushy.

4 Transfer the sorbet to a food processor and process to break up the ice crystals. Put the egg white in a small bowl and lightly whisk with a fork until frothy, then mix it into the sorbet.

5 Pour the sorbet into a plastic or metal container, cover, and freeze for 3–4 hours, or until firm. Let soften at room temperature for 10–15 minutes before serving. Eat within a week of freezing.

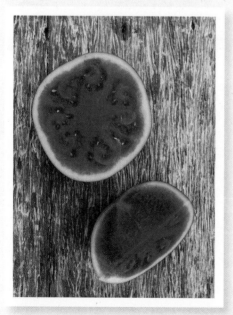

WONDERFUL WATERMELON

Watermelon contains 90 percent water, making it good for rehydrating the body. Unlike alcohol or caffeine, it is gentle on the kidneys. Choose the deepest red-flesh melon you can find for greater amounts of the carotenoid pigment lycopene, which is important for its antioxidant properties and cardiovascular health.

PER SERVING: 210 CAL | 0.7G FAT | TRACE SAT FAT | 52.4G CARBS | 44G SUGARS | TRACE SALT | 4.9G FIBER | 2.9G PROTEIN

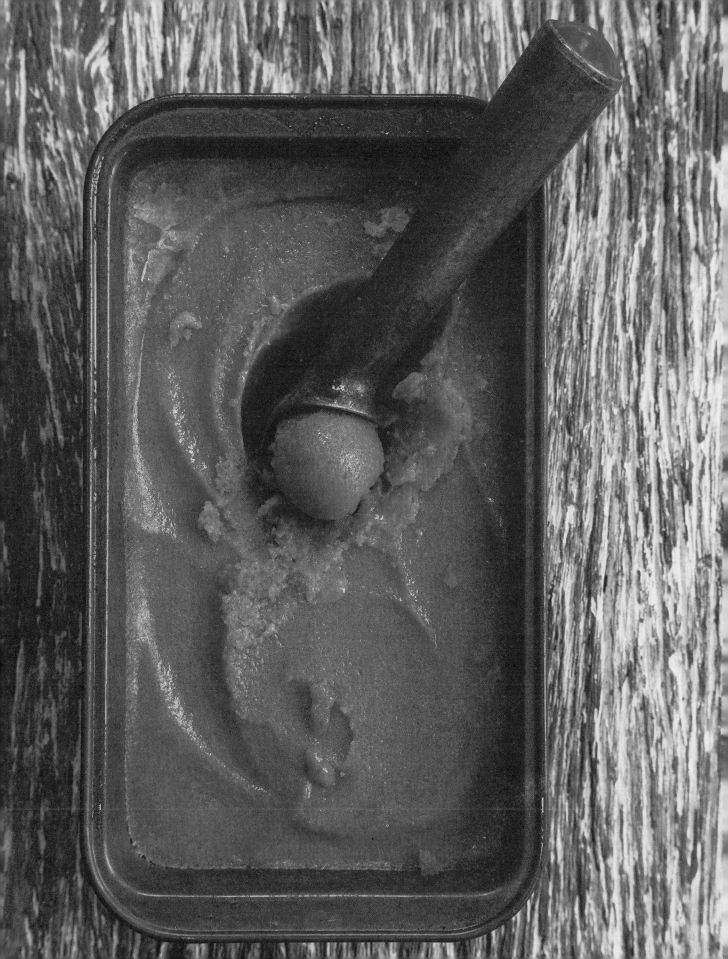

FRUIT COCKTAIL ICE POPS

This is a wonderful way to capture the essence of summer, with the flavors and vibrant colors of ripe, juicy peaches, strawberries, and kiwis.

MAKES: 8 ICE POPS
PREP: 15 MINS   COOK: 12 MINS   FREEZE: 6 HOURS

2½ tablespoons superfine or granulated sugar
¼ cup water
7 ounces strawberries, hulled
2 small peaches, peeled, pitted and coarsely chopped
(or 2 cups drained canned peaches)
4 large kiwis, peeled and coarsely chopped

1 Put the sugar and water into a small saucepan and cook over low heat, stirring, for 5–6 minutes, or until all the sugar has dissolved. Increase the heat to high until the mixture comes to a boil, then reduce the heat to medium and simmer for 3–4 minutes. Let cool completely.

2 Put the strawberries into a food processor or blender and process until pureed. Stir in one-third of the sugar syrup. Pour the mixture into eight ½-cup ice pop molds. Freeze for 2 hours, or until firm.

3 When the strawberry mixture is frozen, put the peaches into the food processor or blender and process until pureed. Stir in half of the remaining sugar syrup. Pour this over the frozen strawberry mixture. Insert the ice pop sticks and freeze for 2 hours, or until firm.

4 When the peach mixture is frozen, put the kiwis into the food processor or blender and process until pureed. Stir in the remaining sugar syrup. Pour this over the frozen peach mixture and freeze for 2 hours, or until firm.

5 To unmold the ice pops, dip the frozen molds into warm water for a few seconds and gently release the pops while holding the sticks.

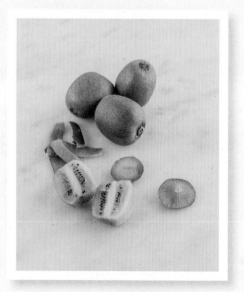

COOL KIWI

Kiwis are a good source of fiber and vitamins A, C, and K and are rich in potassium and folate.

PER ICE POP: 57 CAL | 0.3G FAT | TRACE SAT FAT | 14G CARBS | 11.1G SUGARS | TRACE SALT | 2G FIBER | 0.8G PROTEIN

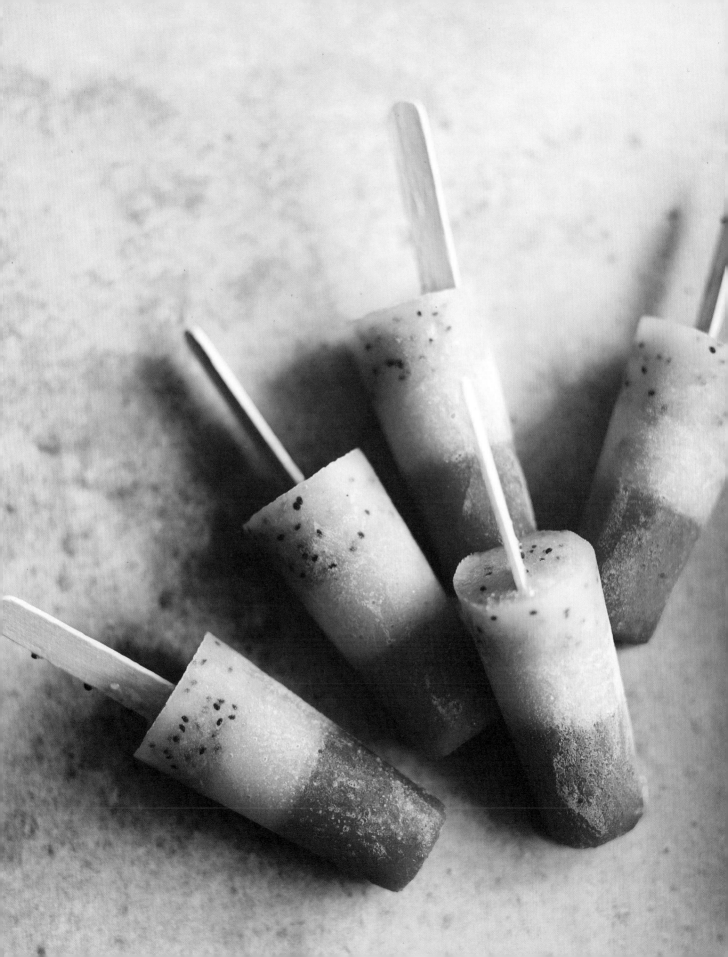

INDEX

almonds 106
   broiled peaches and nectarines 114
   fruity granola cups 34
   honey and blueberry bars 71
   skinny banana split sundaes 106
   warm walnut and orange cake 108
apples 11
   apple and seed muesli 33
   cranberry and red cabbage coleslaw 62
   fruity granola cups 34
   jumbo carrot cake cookies 26
   raw sprouts and seeds supersalad 98
apricots 11, 114
   broiled peaches and nectarines 114
   jumbo carrot cake cookies 26
   raw sprouts and seeds supersalad 98
   warm walnut and orange cake 108
arugula 11
   beef stir-fry 74
   ceviche 46
   risotto primavera 90
asparagus: risotto primavera 90
avocados 14, 67
   avocado and fruit juice 42
   guacamole dip 67
   jerk chicken with papaya and avocado
      salsa 78
   supergreen salad 60

bananas 14, 28
   banana, goji, and hazelnut bread 28
   skinny banana split sundaes 106
barley 12
   barley porridge with broiled papaya
      and peaches 30
beef
   beef stir-fry 74
   stuffed red peppers 94
beets 11, 58
   beet burgers in buns 93
   red beet hash 20
   roasted beet and squash salad 58
bell peppers 11, 50
   beef stir-fry 74
   black bean and quinoa burritos 97
   eggs in red pepper and tomato sauce 22
   stuffed red peppers 94
   sweet red pepper and tomato soup 50
black bean and quinoa burritos 97
blueberries 11, 112
   avocado and fruit juice 42
   creamy coconut and mango quinoa 112
   fruity granola cups 34
   honey and blueberry bars 71
   summer berry sponge cakes 110

yogurt with blueberries, honey, and
   nuts 38
Brazil nuts 108
   cinnamon pancakes with tropical fruit
      salad 24
   power balls 68
   warm walnut and orange cake 108
broccoli 11, 60, 86
   gingered salmon with stir-fried
      kale 86
   supergreen salad 60
buckwheat 33
   apple and seed muesli 33
butternut squash 11
   roasted beet and squash salad 58
   spicy roasted turkey 80

cabbage 11
   cranberry and red cabbage coleslaw 62
carrots 11, 26
   beet burgers in buns 93
   cranberry and red cabbage coleslaw 62
   jumbo carrot cake cookies 26
   lentil and spinach soup 48
   risotto primavera 90
   spicy roasted turkey 80
   Vietnamese tofu and noodle salad 56
cauliflower 11
   cranberry and red cabbage coleslaw 62
   spicy roasted turkey 80
celery: lentil and spinach soup 48
cheese 8
   black bean and quinoa burritos 97
   broiled peaches and nectarines 114
   risotto primavera 90
   shrimp-filled baked sweet potatoes 52
cherries: chocolate, fruit, and nut
   bark 104
chia seeds 12, 78
   jerk chicken with papaya and avocado
      salsa 78
chicken: jerk chicken with papaya and
   avocado salsa 78
chickpeas: stuffed red peppers 94
chocolate 14, 102
   chocolate, cinnamon, and vanilla custard
      desserts 102
   chocolate, fruit, and nut bark 104
   power balls 68
   skinny banana split sundaes 106
coconut
   broiled salmon with mango and lime
      salsa 88
   creamy coconut and mango quinoa 112
   power balls 68

corn kernels: shrimp-filled baked sweet
   potatoes 52
cottage cheese: shrimp-filled baked
   sweet potatoes 52
couscous 12
cranberries 11, 62, 116
   cranberry and raspberry gelatin 116
   cranberry and red cabbage coleslaw 62

dates 12, 68
   apple and seed muesli 33
   power balls 68
dried beans see legumes

edamame
   tangy turkey meatballs with edamame 82
   Vietnamese tofu and noodle salad 56
eggs 11, 24
   chocolate, cinnamon, and vanilla custard
      desserts 102
   cinnamon pancakes with tropical fruit
      salad 24
   eggs in red pepper and tomato sauce 22
   red beet hash 20

farro: roasted beet and squash salad 58
fennel: quinoa salad with fennel and
   orange 54
fish and seafood 12
   broiled salmon with mango and lime
      salsa 88
   broiled trout stuffed with spinach and
      mushrooms 85
   ceviche 46
   gingered salmon with stir-fried kale 86
   shrimp-filled baked sweet potatoes 52
flaxseed 12, 34
   fruity granola cups 34
   jumbo carrot cake cookies 26
   power balls 68
flours 12
fromage blanc: strawberry breakfast dip 37
frozen foods 16

garlic 14, 74
   beef stir-fry 74
   eggs in red pepper and tomato sauce 22
   gingered salmon with stir-fried kale 86
   guacamole dip 67
   lentil and spinach soup 48
   pork medallions with pomegranate salad 76
   risotto primavera 90
   sweet red pepper and tomato soup 50
goji berries 11
   banana, goji, and hazelnut bread 28

fruity granola cups 34
power balls 68
grapefruit 11, 46
ceviche 46
cinnamon pancakes with tropical fruit
salad 24
green tea 14
green tea fruit salad 120

hazelnuts 104
apple and seed muesli 33
banana, goji, and hazelnut bread 28
chocolate, fruit, and nut bark 104
healthy diet 8
hemp seeds 12
herring 12, 88
honey 14, 71
barley porridge with broiled papaya and
peaches 30
broiled peaches and nectarines 114
broiled salmon with mango and lime
salsa 88
chocolate, cinnamon, and vanilla custard
desserts 102
green tea fruit salad 120
honey and blueberry bars 71
yogurt with blueberries, honey, and
nuts 38

Jerusalem artichokes 14, 20
red beet hash 20

kale 11, 40, 60
gingered salmon with stir-fried kale 86
mango and kale juice 40
pork medallions with pomegranate
salad 76
supergreen salad 60
kiwis 11, 124
fruit cocktail ice pops 124
green tea fruit salad 120

leeks 14, 90
gingered salmon with stir-fried kale 86
risotto primavera 90
legumes 12
lentil and spinach soup 48
stuffed red peppers 94
lemons
pork medallions with pomegranate
salad 76
quinoa salad with fennel and orange 54
raw sprouts and seeds supersalad 98
tangy turkey meatballs with edamame 82
lentils 12, 48
lentil and spinach soup 48
stuffed red peppers 94
limes 46
black bean and quinoa burritos 97
broiled salmon with mango and lime
salsa 88
ceviche 46
creamy coconut and mango quinoa 112
guacamole dip 67

raspberry and watermelon sorbet 122
shrimp-filled baked sweet potatoes 52
supergreen salad 60

maca 16
barley porridge with broiled papaya and
peaches 30
power balls 68
mackerel 12, 88
mangoes 11
broiled salmon with mango and lime
salsa 88
cinnamon pancakes with tropical fruit
salad 24
creamy coconut and mango quinoa 112
green tea fruit salad 120
mango and kale juice 40
shrimp-filled baked sweet potatoes 52
maple syrup
fruity granola cups 34
jumbo carrot cake cookies 26
power balls 68
millet
apple and seed muesli 33
beet burgers in buns 93
mint 94
green tea fruit salad 120
stuffed red peppers 94
tangy turkey meatballs with edamame 82
mushrooms
beef stir-fry 74
broiled trout stuffed with spinach and
mushrooms 85

nectarines
broiled peaches and nectarines 114
strawberry breakfast dip 37
noodles: Vietnamese tofu and noodle salad 56
nuts 12
apple and seed muesli 33
banana, goji, and hazelnut bread 28
beet burgers in buns 93
broiled peaches and nectarines 114
chocolate, fruit, and nut bark 104
cinnamon pancakes with tropical fruit
salad 24
cranberry and red cabbage coleslaw 62
fruity granola cups 34
green tea fruit salad 120
honey and blueberry bars 71
jumbo carrot cake cookies 26
pork medallions with pomegranate salad 76
power balls 68
raw sprouts and seeds supersalad 98
skinny banana split sundaes 106
warm walnut and orange cake 108
yogurt with blueberries, honey, and
nuts 38

oats 12
barley porridge with broiled papaya and
peaches 30
fruity granola cups 34
jumbo carrot cake cookies 26

oils 8
onions
eggs in red pepper and tomato sauce 22
lentil and spinach soup 48
sweet red pepper and tomato soup 50
tangy turkey meatballs with edamame 82
oranges 42, 46
avocado and fruit juice 42
gingered salmon with stir-fried kale 86
jumbo carrot cake cookies 26
quinoa salad with fennel and orange 54
warm walnut and orange cake 108

papayas 11, 30
barley porridge with broiled papaya and
peaches 30
green tea fruit salad 120
jerk chicken with papaya and avocado
salsa 78
peaches
barley porridge with broiled papaya and
peaches 30
broiled peaches and nectarines 114
fruit cocktail ice pops 124
pears 11
green tea fruit salad 120
peas
beef stir-fry 74
tangy turkey meatballs with edamame 82
Vietnamese tofu and noodle salad 56
pineapple: cinnamon pancakes with tropical
fruit salad 24
pistachios: green tea fruit salad 120
pomegranates 11, 76
green tea fruit salad 120
pork medallions with pomegranate
salad 76
pork medallions with pomegranate salad 76
preparing fruits and vegetables 7
pumpkin seeds 12
apple and seed muesli 33
fruity granola cups 34
raw sprouts and seeds supersalad 98
supergreen salad 60
pumpkins 11

quinoa 12, 54
black bean and quinoa burritos 97
creamy coconut and mango quinoa 112
honey and blueberry bars 71
quinoa salad with fennel and
orange 54

raspberries 11, 110
cranberry and raspberry gelatin 116
raspberry and watermelon sorbet 122
summer berry sponge cakes 110
red onions
black bean and quinoa burritos 97
ceviche 46
jerk chicken with papaya and avocado
salsa 78
red beet hash 20
stuffed red peppers 94

rice 12, 82
    honey and blueberry bars 71
    risotto primavera 90
    roasted beet and squash salad 58
    tangy turkey meatballs with edamame 82

salmon 12, 88
    broiled salmon with mango and lime
        salsa 88
    gingered salmon with stir-fried kale 86
salt consumption 8
sardines 12, 88
scallions 52
    beef stir-fry 74
    broiled trout stuffed with spinach and
        mushrooms 85
    quinoa salad with fennel and orange 54
    shrimp-filled baked sweet potatoes 52
sea bass: ceviche 46
seeds 12
    apple and seed muesli 33
    eggs in red pepper and tomato sauce 22
    fruity granola cups 34
    jerk chicken with papaya and avocado
        salsa 78
    jumbo carrot cake cookies 26
    mango and kale juice 40
    power balls 68
    raw sprouts and seeds supersalad 98
    spicy roasted turkey 80
    supergreen salad 60
    Vietnamese tofu and noodle salad 56
seed sprouts 14, 98
    cranberry and red cabbage coleslaw 62
    raw sprouts and seeds supersalad 98
sesame seeds 12
    mango and kale juice 40
    power balls 68
    raw sprouts and seeds super salad 98
    spicy roasted turkey 80
    supergreen salad 60
    Vietnamese tofu and noodle salad 56
shrimp-filled baked sweet potatoes 52
snacks 8, 16

snow peas
    beef stir-fry 74
    Vietnamese tofu and noodle salad 56
sodium and salt 8
soy 12, 14
    see also edamame; tofu
spinach 11, 60
    broiled trout stuffed with spinach and
        mushrooms 85
    ceviche 46
    jerk chicken with papaya and avocado
        salsa 78
    lentil and spinach soup 48
    risotto primavera 90
    supergreen salad 60
spirulina 16
sprouting seeds see seed sprouts
strawberries 11, 37, 119
    avocado and fruit juice 42
    fruit cocktail ice pops 124
    fruity granola cups 34
    strawberries with balsamic vinegar 119
    strawberry breakfast dip 37
    summer berry sponge cakes 110
sugar consumption 8
sunflower seeds 12
    apple and seed muesli 33
    fruity granola cups 34
    power balls 68
    raw sprouts and seeds supersalad 98
    spicy roasted turkey 80
    supergreen salad 60
sweet potatoes 11, 64
    red beet hash 20
    shrimp-filled baked sweet potatoes 52
    spicy roasted turkey 80
    sweet potato fries 64
Swiss chard 11
    Vietnamese tofu and noodle salad 56

tofu 14, 56
    Vietnamese tofu and noodle salad 56
tomatoes 11, 22
    black bean and quinoa burritos 97

broiled trout stuffed with spinach and
    mushrooms 85
eggs in red pepper and tomato sauce 22
lentil and spinach soup 48
shrimp-filled baked sweet potatoes 52
stuffed red peppers 94
sweet red pepper and tomato soup 50
trout 12, 85
    broiled trout stuffed with spinach and
        mushrooms 85
    ceviche 46
tuna 12
turkey 8, 14, 80
    spicy roasted turkey 80
    tangy turkey meatballs with edamame 82

walnuts 93
    beet burgers in buns 93
    cranberry and red cabbage coleslaw 62
    pork medallions with pomegranate salad 76
    raw sprouts and seeds supersalad 98
    warm walnut and orange cake 108
watercress 11
    beef stir-fry 74
    ceviche 46
    risotto primavera 90
watermelon 11, 122
    green tea fruit salad 120
    raspberry and watermelon sorbet 122
wheat berries 12
    pork medallions with pomegranate salad 76
wheatgrass 16
whole grains 12

yogurt 11, 38
    beet burgers in buns 93
    chocolate, cinnamon, and vanilla custard
        desserts 102
    fruity granola cups 34
    summer berry sponge cakes 110
    yogurt with blueberries, honey, and nuts 38

zucchini
    beet burgers in buns 93
    risotto primavera 90

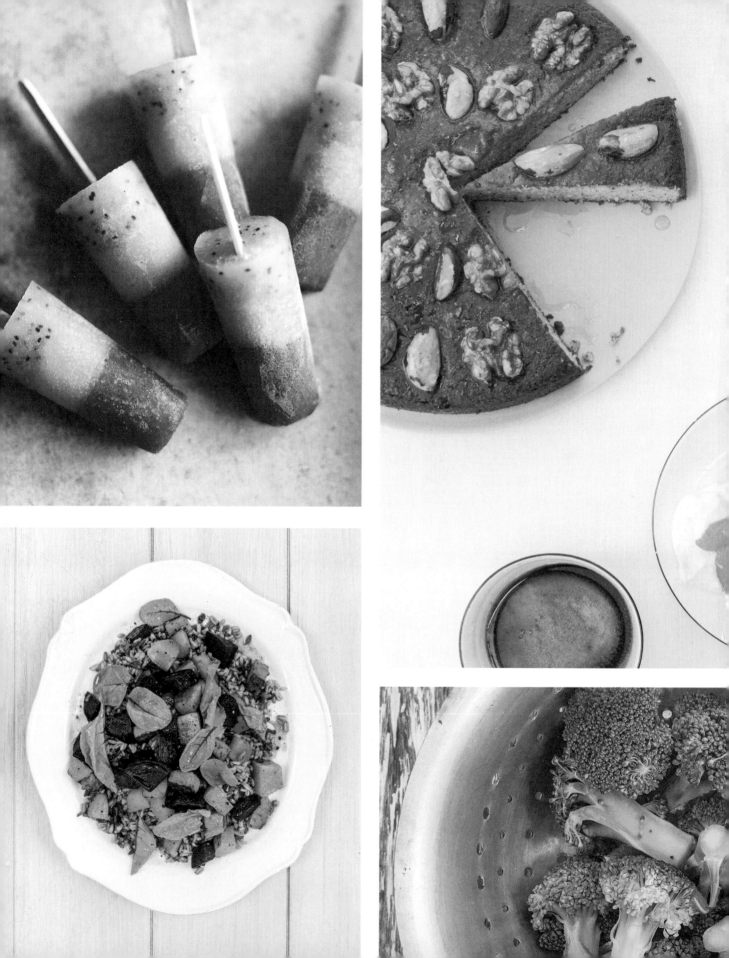